# ASSESSING HEALTH OUTCOMES AMONG VETERANS OF PROJECT SHAD

## (SHIPBOARD HAZARD AND DEFENSE)

Committee on Shipboard Hazard and Defense II (SHAD II)

Board on the Health of Select Populations

Institute of Medicine

*The National Academies of*
SCIENCES · ENGINEERING · MEDICINE

THE NATIONAL ACADEMIES PRESS
*Washington, DC*
**www.nap.edu**

**THE NATIONAL ACADEMIES PRESS 500 Fifth Street, NW Washington, DC 20001**

This activity was supported by Task Order No. 2 under Contract No. VA241-P-2024 from the Department of Veterans Affairs, with additional support from the National Academy of Sciences and the National Academy of Medicine. Any opinions, findings, conclusions, or recommendations expressed in this publication do not necessarily reflect the views of any organization or agency that provided support for the project.

International Standard Book Number-13: 978-0-309-38071-3
International Standard Book Number-10: 0-309-38071-5

Additional copies of this report are available for sale from the National Academies Press, 500 Fifth Street, NW, Keck 360, Washington, DC 20001; (800) 624-6242 or (202) 334-3313; http://www.nap.edu.



Printed in the United States of America

Suggested citation: National Academies of Sciences, Engineering, and Medicine. 2016. *Assessing health outcomes among veterans of Project SHAD (Shipboard Hazard and Defense)*. Washington, DC: The National Academies Press.

*The National Academies of*

SCIENCES · ENGINEERING · MEDICINE

The **National Academy of Sciences** was established in 1863 by an Act of Congress, signed by President Lincoln, as a private, nongovernmental institution to advise the nation on issues related to science and technology. Members are elected by their peers for outstanding contributions to research. Dr. Ralph J. Cicerone is president.

The **National Academy of Engineering** was established in 1964 under the charter of the National Academy of Sciences to bring the practices of engineering to advising the nation. Members are elected by their peers for extraordinary contributions to engineering. Dr. C. D. Mote, Jr., is president.

The **National Academy of Medicine** (formerly the Institute of Medicine) was established in 1970 under the charter of the National Academy of Sciences to advise the nation on medical and health issues. Members are elected by their peers for distinguished contributions to medicine and health. Dr. Victor J. Dzau is president.

The three Academies work together as the **National Academies of Sciences, Engineering, and Medicine** to provide independent, objective analysis and advice to the nation and conduct other activities to solve complex problems and inform public policy decisions. The Academies also encourage education and research, recognize outstanding contributions to knowledge, and increase public understanding in matters of science, engineering, and medicine.

Learn more about the National Academies of Sciences, Engineering, and Medicine at **www.national-academies.org.**

## COMMITTEE ON SHIPBOARD HAZARD AND DEFENSE II (SHAD II)

**DAVID J. TOLLERUD** (*Chair*), Professor and Chair, Department of Environmental and Occupational Health Sciences, University of Louisville School of Public Health and Information Sciences
**JOSEPH A. BOSCARINO,** Senior Scientist, Center for Health Research, Geisinger Clinic, Danville, Pennsylvania
**LINDA A. MCCAULEY,** Professor and Dean, Nell Hodgson Woodruff School of Nursing, Emory University
**THOMAS E. MCKONE,** Senior Staff Scientist and Deputy Division Director, Lawrence Berkeley National Laboratory
**KENNETH R. STILL,** Scientific Director and Senior Toxicology and Industrial Hygiene Consultant, Occupational Toxicology Associates, Inc., Lake Oswego, Oregon, and Adjunct Assistant Professor, Portland State University, School of Community Health, College of Urban and Public Affairs, Portland, Oregon
**BETH A. VIRNIG,** Professor and Senior Associate Dean for Academic Affairs and Research, University of Minnesota School of Public Health
**YILIANG ZHU,** Professor, Department of Epidemiology and Biostatistics, College of Public Health, and Professor, Internal Medicine, Morsani College of Medicine, University of South Florida

*Consultants*
**DANIEL H. FREEMAN, JR.,** Professor Emeritus of Preventive Medicine and Community Health, University of Texas Medical Branch at Galveston
**CYNTHIA C. JOHNSON,** Nosologist, Richmond, Virginia
**ALFRED K. MBAH,** Assistant Professor of Biostatistics and Epidemiology, University of South Florida
**JAMES E. QUINN,** Commander, U.S. Navy, Retired

*IOM Staff*
**LOIS JOELLENBECK,** Study Director
**HARRIET CRAWFORD,** IT Project Manager
**REINE HOMAWOO,** Programmer/Analyst
**DWAYNE BELL,** Programmer/Analyst (through June 2015)
**HEATHER YOUNG,** Biostatistician (through November 2014)
**JANE DURCH,** Senior Program Officer
**JON SANDERS,** Program Associate (through January 2015)
**ASHLEY MAYO,** Intern (Summer 2012, 2013)
**JULIE WILTSHIRE,** Financial Associate
**FREDERICK ERDTMANN,** Director, Board on the Health of Select Populations

# Reviewers

This report has been reviewed in draft form by individuals chosen for their diverse perspectives and technical expertise. The purpose of this independent review is to provide candid and critical comments that will assist the institution in making its published report as sound as possible and to ensure that the report meets institutional standards for objectivity, evidence, and responsiveness to the study charge. The review comments and draft manuscript remain confidential to protect the integrity of the deliberative process. We wish to thank the following individuals for their review of this report:

**David B. Allison,** University of Alabama at Birmingham
**Joel Greenhouse,** Carnegie Mellon University
**David G. Hoel,** Exponent
**Howard M. Kipen,** Rutgers School of Public Health
**Kenneth W. Kizer,** University of California, Davis, School of Medicine and Betty Irene Moore School of Nursing
**Nan M. Laird,** School of Public Health, Harvard University
**Raphael C. Lee,** The University of Chicago
**David A. Macys,** Oak Harbor, Washington
**Robert B. Wallace,** University of Iowa College of Public Health

Although the reviewers listed above have provided many constructive comments and suggestions, they were not asked to endorse the conclusions or recommendations nor did they see the final draft of the report before its release. The review of this report was overseen by **Stephen E. Fienberg,** Carnegie Mellon University, and **George W. Rutherford,** University of California, San Francisco. They were responsible for making certain that an independent examination of this report was carried out in accordance with institutional procedures and that all review comments were carefully considered. Responsibility for the final content of this report rests entirely with the authoring committee and the institution.

# Preface

When the secret Project Shipboard Hazard and Defense (SHAD) testing program was made public in 2000, veterans reasonably wondered what impact their involvement in the testing might have had on their health.

Following the release of the first Institute of Medicine (IOM) SHAD report in 2007, Congress requested that the IOM undertake a new epidemiological study of the potential long-term health effects of participation in the SHAD testing. Our committee, with expertise in epidemiology, occupational health, biostatistics, exposure assessment, toxicology, and Vietnam veterans' health issues, was convened to examine this question, a role the committee took very seriously. Our careful review of published scientific literature on the agents, simulants, tracers, and decontaminants used in the tests, led us to formulate hypotheses on health effects that might be associated with exposure to six of these substances. We also undertook exploratory analyses to ensure that unanticipated associations would not be overlooked.

Our task was challenging because of the passage of time since the tests, and because many of the documents related to the tests remain classified. Our requests for declassification of additional documents were not approved. Using the limited information available in redacted reports on these tests, the committee evaluated exposure opportunities that test participants may have had.

The study faced other challenges as well. Protecting the security of the data used in the study was, of course, of high importance to the committee and to the Department of Veterans Affairs (VA). Meeting those obligations made it necessary to work within the VA information technology system, and this posed a series of requirements that significantly delayed all aspects of our data processing and analysis. These delays also limited the depth of the data analysis that could be accomplished over the life of the study. The committee was successful in performing an extensive review of the mortality data, but analysis of the morbidity data was more limited.

In the course of our efforts, the committee benefited from the help of several organizations and individuals. We are particularly grateful to the veterans of SHAD testing who gave their time and efforts to helping to orient us to our task at the start of the study. SHAD veteran Jack Alderson was tireless in providing background to the study staff and serving as a liaison to other veterans. We appreciated use of the VA Informatics and Computing Infrastructure system to host and access data; that arrangement made completion of the study possible under difficult circumstances. We are grateful for the considerable help we received from VA in using the system, particularly John Quinn, Susan Hickey, Jeffrey Scehnet, and their team. We are grateful as well to Rebecca Crawford, Gayle Lyke, Wendi Dick, Loren Erickson, Octavia Dixon, and Terry Walters who worked with us at the VA Office of Public Health. At and through the Department of Defense, we received assistance from Michael Kilpatrick, Dee Morris, Arnold Dupuy, Nathan Pawlicki, Anthony Lee, Dupont Durst, and Kenneth Gritton. We also appreciate the help of Timothy Daly, formerly of Congressman Mike Thompson's office, and John Driscoll, of Congressman Jared Huffman's office. We appreciated the input and extensive background materials from Rick Weidman, Bernard Edelman, and Thomas Berger of the Vietnam Veterans of America.

I am also very grateful to my fellow committee members, volunteers who have shown great commitment to the effort, giving without complaint an additional two years of their time and expertise beyond what was initially anticipated. I also thank consultants Dan Freeman, Alfred Mbah, and James

Quinn, who made important contributions of expertise and time. On behalf of the committee, I commend the expert and tireless work of the IOM staff, including study director Lois Joellenbeck; the data team of Harriet Crawford, Reine Homawoo, and Dwayne Bell; Jane Durch, Julie Wiltshire, Andrea Cohen, Greta Gorman, Jon Sanders, and Ashley Mayo. We also appreciate the assistance and support of David Butler, Director of the Medical Follow-up Agency; Frederick Erdtmann, Director of the Board on the Health of Select Populations; and Clyde Behney, Executive Director, Institute of Medicine.

David J. Tollerud, *Chair*
Committee on Shipboard Hazard and Defense II

# Contents

# Abbreviations and Acronyms

| | |
|---|---|
| AChE | acetylcholinesterase |
| AIHA | American Industrial Hygiene Association |
| ARR | adjusted rate ratio |
| ATS | Academy of Toxicological Sciences |
| ATSDR | Agency for Toxic Substances and Disease Registry |
| | |
| BG | *Bacillus globigii* |
| BPL | betapropiolactone |
| | |
| CAS | Chemical Abstracts Service |
| CB | *Coxiella burnetii* |
| CBRN | chemical, biological, radiological, and nuclear |
| CCRIS | Chemical Carcinogenesis Research Information System |
| CDC | Centers for Disease Control and Prevention |
| CdS | cadmium sulfide |
| CI | confidence interval |
| CIDRAP | Center for Infectious Disease Research and Policy |
| CLE | confocal laser endomicroscopy |
| CMS | Centers for Medicare & Medicaid Services |
| CNS | central nervous system |
| COPD | chronic obstructive pulmonary disease |
| CRI | Center for Research Information |
| | |
| DEP | diethylphthalate |
| DNA | deoxyribonucleic acid |
| DoD | Department of Defense |
| DoN | Department of the Navy |
| DTC | Deseret Test Center |
| DTIC | Defense Technical Information Center |
| | |
| EC | *Escherichia coli* |
| EPA | Environmental Protection Agency |

| | |
|---|---|
| FDR | false discovery rate |
| FOIA | Freedom of Information Act |
| FWER | family-wise error rate |
| | |
| GAO | Government Accountability Office (formerly General Accounting Office) |
| GI | gastrointestinal |
| | |
| HHS | Department of Health and Human Services |
| HR | hazard ratio |
| HSDB | Hazardous Substances Data Bank |
| | |
| IARC | International Agency for Research on Cancer |
| ICD | *International Classification of Diseases* |
| IOM | Institute of Medicine |
| IRIS | Integrated Risk Information System |
| | |
| LT | light tug |
| | |
| m | meter |
| MAA | methyl acetoacetate |
| MCS | mental component summary (of the Short Form 36 Health Survey [SF-36]) |
| MedPAR | Medicare Provider Analysis and Review |
| MFUA | Medical Follow-up Agency |
| mg | milligram |
| MRC | material condition of readiness |
| | |
| NARA | National Archives and Records Administration |
| NDI | National Death Index |
| NIOSH | National Institute for Occupational Safety and Health |
| NMRI | Naval Medical Research Institute |
| NRC | National Research Council |
| NTP | National Toxicology Program |
| | |
| OP | organophosphorus |
| OR | odds ratio |
| OU | *Coxiella burnetti* |
| | |
| PCS | physical component summary (of the SF-36) |
| PL | Public Law |
| PNS | peripheral nervous system |
| PSTS | Project SHAD Technical Staff |
| PTHrP | parathyroid hormone-related protein |
| PVC | polyvinyl chloride |
| | |
| RADS | reactive airways dysfunction syndrome |

| | |
|---|---|
| RR | rate ratio |
| | |
| SAS | Statistical Analysis System |
| SEA | staphylococcal enterotoxin type A |
| SEB | staphylococcal enterotoxin type B |
| SHAD | Shipboard Hazard and Defense |
| SM | *Serratia marcescens* |
| SMR | standardized mortality ratio |
| SQL | Structured Query Language |
| SSA | Social Security Administration |
| STOPS | Shipboard Toxicological Operational Protection System |
| | |
| TCDD | tetrachlorodibenzodioxin |
| TEHP | tris(2-ethylhexyl) phosphate, also known as trioctyl phosphate (TOF) |
| TOF | trioctyl phosphate |
| | |
| UL | *Pasteurella tularensis* |
| | |
| VA | Department of Veterans Affairs |
| VBA | Veterans Benefits Administration |
| VHA | Veterans Health Administration |
| VINCI | VA Informatics and Computing Infrastructure |
| | |
| ZnCdS | zinc cadmium sulfide |
| ZnS | zinc sulfide |

# Summary

Between 1963 and 1969, the U.S. military carried out a series of tests, termed Project SHAD (Shipboard Hazard and Defense), to evaluate the vulnerabilities of U.S. Navy ships to chemical and biological warfare agents. These tests involved use of active chemical and biological agents, simulants, tracers, and decontaminants. Approximately 5,900 military personnel, primarily from the Navy and Marine Corps, are reported to have been included in Project SHAD testing. At the time they were conducted, virtually all aspects of the Project 112/SHAD tests were assigned a security classification of Secret or Top Secret.

In the 1990s some veterans who participated in the SHAD tests expressed concerns to the Department of Veterans Affairs (VA) that their health problems might be the result of exposures in the testing. Congress and VA requested information from the Department of Defense (DoD) to clarify what substances veterans may have been exposed to and when the tests had taken place. In 2002 and 2003 DoD publicly released fact sheets that described each test, identified the participating military units, and named the chemical and biological agents, simulants, decontaminants, and tracers used, but many details about the tests remain classified.

Studies by the Institute of Medicine (IOM) and VA researchers, published in 2007-2009, produced complex results. The IOM study found no difference in all-cause mortality between SHAD veterans and the comparison group, but there was an increased risk of death from heart disease among some SHAD veterans and responses to a 2004 health survey indicated poorer overall physical and mental health among the SHAD participants. The VA study found an increase in all-cause mortality among the SHAD veterans that was due primarily to heart disease.

In response to continuing concerns, Congress in 2010 requested an additional IOM study (SHAD II). The SHAD II study, reported on here, expanded on the previous IOM work by making use of additional years of follow up and some analysis of diagnostic data from Medicare and the VA health care system. In finding no overall differences in all-cause mortality between SHAD participants and comparison groups, the SHAD II analysis agreed with the results of the previous IOM study. However, it differed in that, with an additional 7 years of follow up, it did not find an elevation in heart disease mortality. Indications of an increased risk of heart disease in the crew of the USS *George Eastman*, one of the exposure groups examined, did not attain statistical significance after adjustment for the multiple comparisons carried out in the analysis. The SHAD II analysis found no clear differences in degree of illness between SHAD participants and the comparison group. This result was consistent with the absence of differences in self-reported hospitalizations noted in SHAD I, but not in accord with the SHAD I survey responses that indicated overall worse health among SHAD veterans.

## THE SHAD II STUDY

The Caregivers and Veterans Omnibus Health Services Act of 2010 (PL 111-163) requested that the IOM conduct a new epidemiological study of the potential long-term health effects of participation in the SHAD testing. The charge to the Committee on Shipboard Hazard and Defense (SHAD) II appears in Box S-1.

The intent of Project SHAD was to evaluate operational characteristics of ships and protective and dissemination equipment as well as the behavior of test agents in marine environments. Although exposure samples (e.g., gargle samples or chemical dosimeters on clothing) were obtained from the men present during a few tests, the purpose of the SHAD tests was not study the health of the participants.

The SHAD tests involved use of active chemical and biological agents, simulants, tracers, and decontaminants. The active chemical and biological agents were potential weapons and known to be debilitating or even fatal in the short term to unprotected personnel. The simulants were substances that shared certain chemical or biological characteristics of the active agents but were considered at the time to be relatively safe to use. For example, *Bacillus globigii* (BG) has been used for many years as a simulant for the aerosol behavior of *Bacillus anthracis*, which causes the disease anthrax. Tracers were substances used to track the movement of test agents or simulants.

### Approach to the Study

The committee's interest was in evaluating whether the long-term health of SHAD veterans has been adversely affected by their exposures during SHAD testing. Specifically, the committee sought to determine (1) whether participation in SHAD tests that used certain agents, simulants, tracers, or decontaminants is associated with differences in specific long-term health effects, as manifested in greater risk of mortality or morbidity (hypothesis-based analysis); and

**BOX S-1**
**Study Charge**

An ad hoc committee of experts in conjunction with the Institute of Medicine's (IOM's) Medical Follow-up Agency (MFUA) staff will conduct an epidemiological study comparing the health status of the SHAD veterans with a comparison population. This study will build on knowledge gained from a prior study (Long-Term Health Effects of Participation in Project SHAD) conducted by MFUA staff between 2003 and 2007. The SHAD II study will use the established SHAD participants list and the comparison population list of individuals determined from the prior study.

As part of the data collection process, the committee will plan and conduct an initial workshop to receive suggestions and input from SHAD veterans about their experiences so that the study can be informed by new insights from this group.

Following the completion of the study, the committee will author an IOM report summarizing the approach and findings of this study.

If the results of this SHAD II study indicate a difference in outcome between the SHAD participants and the comparison population, or if the study finds new information that would warrant new research avenues, MFUA will be prepared to conduct additional research as appropriate.

(2) whether Project SHAD participants were at increased risk of mortality or morbidity across a broad range of standard diagnostic categories (exploratory analysis) compared with veterans who served on similar ships or in similar units that did not participate in the SHAD tests. "Long-term" was taken to mean persisting or recurring conditions as well as those appearing several years or more after exposure.

The SHAD II study was a retrospective cohort design. The study population consisted of men identified by DoD from ship logs and personnel diaries as having been present during some portion of at least one SHAD test. To assemble the comparison population, ships and Marine Corps units that participated in SHAD tests were matched, to the extent possible, with a ship (or unit) of a similar class, crew complement, operating area, and home port at the time of the SHAD test. The crew members of the five light tug boats (9-12 men per boat) could be identified for only one of the several tests that they participated in, and no comparison vessels could be named. Identification of the study population is described in greater detail in Chapters 2 and 3, and a list of all ships and units from which the study population was drawn is provided in Appendix E.

## Generating Hypotheses Concerning SHAD Exposures

Using existing summaries of older literature and a review of the scientific literature published in 2000 or later, the committee examined information on the potential health effects from exposure to the substances used in the SHAD tests. On the basis of this review, the committee generated hypotheses about health outcomes that might be associated with six of the test substances (see Table S-1) and used them as a way to focus portions of its analysis.

**TABLE S-1** Hypotheses to Be Tested Concerning Certain Substances Used in SHAD Testing and Adverse Health Outcomes

| Substance | Use in SHAD Test | Health Outcome Hypothesized |
|---|---|---|
| *Coxiella burnetii* | Biological agent | Chronic hepatitis<br>Endocarditis<br>Fatigue syndrome<br>Osteomyelitis<br>Vascular infection |
| *Escherichia coli* | Biological simulant | Irritable bowel syndrome |
| Staphylococcal enterotoxin type B[a] | Biological agent | Asthma<br>Graves' disease<br>Multiple sclerosis<br>Rheumatoid arthritis |
| Sarin | Chemical agent | Neurological effects (central nervous system)<br>Neurological effects (peripheral nervous system)<br>Neurological effects (hearing loss)<br>Psychological symptoms |
| Betapropiolactone | Decontaminant | Cancer (any type) |
| Zinc cadmium sulfide | Tracer | Chronic kidney disease<br>Lung cancer |

[a] Because the individuals who served on the vessels involved in testing staphylococcal enterotoxin type B were not identified, the committee could not test the hypotheses generated for this agent.

## Exposure

The nature of SHAD veterans' potential exposures vary. The SHAD tests involved at least 19 different vessels and seven Marine Corps units in 21 tests that used at least 16 different test substances (alone or in combination) over a period of 7 years. Each test included multiple trials (ranging from as few as 5 to as many as 31), and the participating ships and test substances could vary from trial to trial within a test. For ships that participated in multiple tests, crew members could change from test to test. Approximately 69 percent of the SHAD participants (4,050 men) were in only one test. The remainder participated in from two to seven tests.

### *Exposure Groups*

Substance-specific exposure groups were created where possible for the substances for which hypotheses regarding health outcomes were formulated. Also created were three broad exposure groups based on the substances used in the SHAD tests: (1) any biological substance; (2) any chemical substance, except trioctyl phosphate (TOF); and (3) any decontaminant. These exposure groups are not mutually exclusive; a member of the study population might be included in any or all of them.

Analyses were also conducted of three subgroups with distinctive experiences: (1) the crew of the USS *George Eastman*, a specially outfitted ship involved in multiple tests, including some with live agents; (2) members of the Project SHAD technical staff, including persons with service on the light tugs, who were identified in a roster from January 1965; and (3) participants in Test 69-10, who received unique exposure to TOF. The membership of these groups was largely mutually exclusive.

Special consideration was also given to the crew of the USS *Granville S. Hall*; which served as the laboratory ship for many SHAD tests. The ship's regular crew was supplemented by identified members of the Project SHAD technical staff. For overall analyses, the committee included all *Granville S. Hall* crew members as part of the Project SHAD population. For analyses that addressed specific forms of exposure, the Project SHAD technical staff was considered as potentially exposed and the members of the regular crew were excluded as unexposed.

The comparison group for each of the exposure groups was determined on the basis of the tests in which the exposures occurred, the units in the test that received the specified exposure, and the designated comparison unit for that test.

### *Exposure Opportunities*

Data were compiled on cumulative numbers of exposure events for each of the test substances for each man identified as being present during the test period. For example, a person present on a ship for nine trials in one test and for three trials in another test that used the same substance would be considered to have 12 exposures (9 + 3 = 12) to that substance. Where the size of the exposed group and the variation in the number of potential exposures were considered sufficient, the committee established subgroups to reflect the range of exposure experience (e.g., low, medium, high) among the SHAD participants. Appendix D includes a description of the process used to evaluate the distribution of exposure opportunities and determine the exposure subgroups.

## Data on Health Outcomes

The committee evaluated the causes of deaths in the study population since the 1960s and the diagnoses assigned at hospital and outpatient visits in data from Medicare from 1999 through 2011 and from the VA health system from late 1997 through 2011.

### *Mortality*

Mortality follow-up for SHAD participants began at the date of their first test exposure, and ended on the date of death or December 31, 2011, whichever came first. In addition to the members of the study population known to be dead at the time of the first IOM study, additional deaths were determined through automated matching with records of the Veterans Benefits Administration and records available through Lexis/Nexis. Data on cause of death were obtained from the National Death Index or from death certificates obtained from state vital statistics offices for 91 percent of the members of the study population who were identified as deceased. The underlying cause of death was assigned a code corresponding to the *International Classification of Diseases* (ICD, 9th or 10th revisions).

### *Morbidity*

After leaving military service, some veterans receive medical care from VA facilities, many receive care from clinicians and facilities in the community, and some may receive care from both sources. On reaching age 65, almost all veterans become eligible for Medicare, but some may continue to receive some or all of their care through VA or private insurance. The SHAD II study assessed morbidity through records collected into automated databases as a byproduct of medical care received through VA or under the auspices of Medicare billing. As of December 31, 2011, 83 percent of the study participants assumed alive were 65 years of age or older.

The VA data were derived from multiple datasets held by the Veterans Health Administration (VHA), including Inpatient Encounters, Bed section acute care dataset, Main acute care dataset, Procedure acute care dataset, Surgery acute care dataset, and Event dataset. These files captured overlapping information on inpatient and outpatient encounters.

Medicare enrollment information is provided in the Master Beneficiary Summary File (formerly the Denominator File). Data on diagnoses were derived from the Medicare Provider Analysis and Review (MedPAR) file (hospital stays) and the Outpatient and Carrier files (services provided in non-inpatient facilities and care by physicians). The Medicare data do not include information about care provided to Medicare Managed Care enrollees or care provided outside of the Medicare program. Diagnostic data are available only for conditions for which diagnoses have been recorded as part of a health care claim, and some conditions that could have been diagnosed are not recorded.

## THE STUDY POPULATION

The population for this study was made up of 5,868 Project SHAD participants and 6,753 other veterans who served as the comparison group. Approximately 60 percent of both groups were born in 1937-1946, and about 18 to 19 percent born earlier and 15 to 16 percent born later. Date of birth was unknown for 5.4 percent of SHAD veterans and 8.4 percent of the comparison population. The proportion of personnel who were white was 87 to 88 percent of those whose race was known in participant and comparison groups. In both groups, the majority served in the Navy (86 percent of SHAD veterans and 91 percent of the comparison group) and were enlisted personnel (92 and 93 percent, respectively). Similar proportions of the two groups had evidence from a VA disability application of service in Vietnam or presumed or documented exposure to Agent Orange. The similarity of the two groups on these factors offered some assurance that the two populations were reasonably comparable.

## FINDINGS ON MORTALITY

As of December 31, 2011, approximately 30 percent of both the SHAD veterans and the comparison population had died. Kaplan-Meier survival analysis showed no evidence of statistically significant difference between the participant and comparison groups in the overall number or timing of deaths. When cause of death, grouped by broad ICD categories, was examined using a Cox proportional hazards model that adjusted for age, Project SHAD veterans showed no statistically significant increases in hazard over the comparison population.

### Testing Hypotheses on Exposures

In analyses limited to the SHAD veterans exposed to the five test substances for which it was possible to test the committee's hypotheses regarding health outcomes, no statistically significant differences were seen in all-cause mortality. This held true as well when the enlisted and officer groups were examined separately.

In analyses that examined the specific causes of death identified in the committee's hypotheses, proportional hazards analysis that included adjustment for age and rank found no statistically significant excess risk among SHAD participants for the two exposures (betapropriolactone and zinc cadmium sulfide) for which there were sufficient numbers of cases to pursue the analysis. No significant differences emerged when the enlisted group was examined separately or when the analysis took into account whether the SHAD veterans had a greater or lesser number of exposures to these substances.

### Exploratory Analysis in Subgroups of Special Interest

*All-Cause Mortality*

All-cause mortality among the members of the groups of special interest was not significantly different from that among their comparison groups, and stratifying the groups on the basis of rank (officer and enlisted) resulted in no statistically significant differences. Members of the tug and Project SHAD technical staff subgroup had higher crude mortality when compared to the other members of the crew of the USS *Granville S. Hall* or to the crew of the comparison vessel for the *Granville S. Hall* (external control), but this difference was accounted for by the older age of this subgroup of SHAD veterans.

*Number of Potential Exposures*

For three groups—those exposed to any biological substance, to any chemical substance except TOF, or to any decontaminant—it was possible to assess whether higher or lower numbers of potential exposures influenced mortality risks. Using two or three levels of exposure, depending upon the numbers of people exposed and the distribution of the exposure counts across the group, no significant differences emerged at any level of exposure. This type of dose–response analysis was not feasible for the other exposure groups because of the limited variation within the group in the number of exposure opportunities.

*Cause-Specific Mortality*

When mortality attributed to specific causes was examined, an increase in risk among SHAD participants was seen only in the crew of the USS *George Eastman*, for heart disease mortality. However, when the committee applied a statistical adjustment to take into account the multiple comparisons in the analysis, the result no longer attained statistical significance.

## FINDINGS ON MORBIDITY

Diagnoses noted in records generated as a result of medical care received under the auspices of the Medicare program or through VA were the basis for the assessment of morbidity in the study population. Approximately 55 percent of the SHAD veterans and 52 percent of the comparison population had ever been enrolled in the fee-for-service form of Medicare. Although comparable "enrollment" data are not available for VA health care, the committee found that 40 percent of SHAD veterans and 33 percent of the comparison population had indications of use of inpatient or outpatient care through VA, a statistically significant difference. An increase in use of VA health care among Project SHAD veterans relative to the comparison population was observed beginning in 2002, which is when VA began notifying SHAD veterans of their participation in the previously secret SHAD testing. By 2005, usage of VA health services among SHAD veterans remained higher than that of the comparison population, but the rate of increase in use from year to year became similar in the two groups.

### Overall Morbidity

Overall morbidity was evaluated using median hospital days per person-year of enrollment among Medicare enrollees hospitalized during the study period. Roughly 42 percent of both Project SHAD participant and comparison groups who had been enrolled in Medicare during the study period had a hospitalization during that time. Median hospital days per person-year of enrollment among those hospitalized was slightly lower among Project SHAD participants than the comparison group, but the difference was not statistically significant. Looking at broad categories of disease showed that circulatory disease was the most common diagnosis in the Medicare data in both groups, with approximately 51 percent in each group having such a diagnosis. The proportions receiving diagnoses of other types were also comparable in the two groups. Again in data from VA, the percentages of diagnoses in various categories were not higher in the SHAD veteran group than in the comparison group.

### Testing Hypotheses on Exposures

The committee focused its morbidity analysis on the members of the study population with exposure to the substances for which hypotheses regarding health outcomes were developed. Of those enrolled in Medicare, 41 to 53 percent were hospitalized during the study period. Among those hospitalized, median hospital days per person-year of enrollment were not statistically higher in the SHAD veterans in the exposure groups than in their comparison groups. The results of cause-specific analysis also showed no statistically significant increases in the specific causes of morbidity identified in the committee's hypotheses.

## DISCUSSION

Testimony and other information from SHAD veterans was essential in helping the committee gain a better understanding of the context of the SHAD tests and the experience of those who had been present. The study also benefited from the efforts during the previous IOM study to establish and validate the cohort of Project SHAD test participants from ship logs and diaries. The previous IOM study also provided the unique benefit of a comparison population of military personnel with service more comparable in time and character to that of the SHAD veterans than would typically be found. With nearly 50 years of follow-up since the first SHAD test, the study had an opportunity to assess the mortality experience of the study population across a broad range of causes of death, including those that appear later in life. Similarly, the long follow-up period made it feasible to turn to Medicare data to examine morbidity.

But the study also faced important challenges. The time that has elapsed since the tests took place in the 1960s makes it difficult to account for all the factors beyond the SHAD tests that will have influenced the health of the veterans who participated in the tests. The evidence from VA data that similar proportions of the SHAD veterans and the comparison population appeared to have had service in Vietnam and possible exposure to Agent Orange provides some reassurance that those factors did not have a marked influence on the analysis.

The study was also constrained by the limits of the available documentation. Information on the concentrations of test substances and results from sampling stations largely remains classified. Having access to the classified material in Project SHAD reports might have informed the committee regarding the range of potential exposures for a given unit in a test. However, because the location of individual crew members during tests was also not available, the committee still could not have estimated doses at the individual level, and the statistical analyses would remain those of comparing exposure groups. As a result, the committee does not expect that having the classified information would alter the findings of the analysis. Rosters listing the crews of the tugs were not available except for one early test, preventing testing of one of the a priori hypotheses developed by the committee. The committee also lacked data for explicit exploration of the concerns of certain SHAD veterans about exposure to vaccines against biological warfare agents or exposure to residual radiation from nuclear tests previously conducted in areas of the Pacific Ocean where SHAD tests were also conducted.

Analytical challenges arose from the complexity of the data. While the Medicare data for enrollees over age 65 can be interpreted as providing population-based measures, data from VA are harder to interpret because of the variable criteria for eligibility for and decisions to use these services. But at no time was the entire Project SHAD participant cohort eligible for Medicare. Thus the committee's analysis had to focus on the morbidity of the oldest veterans, who were also the oldest at the time of the testing.

The committee's use of hypotheses generated from the literature provided some focus for the analyses, but in assessing the health status of SHAD participants and the comparison groups for various categories of exposures the committee carried out many statistical tests, increasing the likelihood that statistically significant associations could arise by chance. In some cases the exposure groups were of modest size, which could make it difficult to ascertain any true subtle differences in either mortality or morbidity.

Although the committee was cognizant of the questions raised by veterans and others about the ethics and legality of the SHAD testing, it was not charged with reviewing the merits of the program. Its focus had to be on the scientific question of whether test participation is associated with adverse long-term health effects.

## CONCLUSIONS

Epidemiological studies such as this investigation of health outcomes among veterans of the SHAD tests are complex undertakings requiring substantial time and resources. The committee invested considerable effort in learning about the SHAD tests and in formulating its approaches to data analysis. In the numerous analyses of both the full study population and of several subgroups, the only finding of a seemingly higher risk—of heart disease mortality among the 356 men who served on the USS *George Eastman*—did not attain statistical significance after adjustments for the multiple tests carried out on this group. The vast majority of the analyses showed no evidence of different health outcomes among SHAD veterans relative to the comparison group. The committee recognizes that with the limitations of epidemiological studies these negative findings cannot unequivocally rule out some potential effect from the SHAD testing. However, within the limits of the data available to the committee, the results of the analyses provide no evidence that the health of SHAD veterans overall or those in the exposure groups is significantly different from that of similar veterans who did not participate in these tests.

# 1

# Introduction

In the 1960s the U.S. military carried out a series of tests to evaluate the vulnerabilities of U.S. Navy ships to chemical and biological warfare agents. Termed Project SHAD (Shipboard Hazard and Defense), this effort was a component of Project 112, a larger program that included both land- and sea-based testing as part of a chemical and biological warfare readiness effort by the Department of Defense (DoD) and the military services. Approximately 5,900 military servicemen, primarily from the Navy and Marine Corps, are reported to have been included in Project SHAD testing.

In the 1990s some veterans who participated in the SHAD tests expressed concerns to the Department of Veterans Affairs (VA) that they were experiencing health problems that might be the result of exposures in the testing. Congress and VA requested information from DoD to clarify what substances veterans may have been exposed to and when the tests had taken place. At the time they were conducted, virtually all aspects of the Project 112/SHAD tests were assigned a security classification of Secret or Top Secret, but in 2002 DoD publicly released fact sheets that described each test, identified the participating military units, and named the agents, simulants, decontaminants, and tracers used (DoD, 2015). Some of the fact sheets were revised in 2003 as DoD corrected or supplemented the initial documents.

The health concerns of the SHAD veterans also led to a 2002 request from VA to the Institute of Medicine (IOM) to carry out an epidemiological study of the health of SHAD veterans and a comparison population of veterans who had served on similar ships or in similar units during the same time period. The results of the study, published in 2007 (IOM, 2007) and referred to in the remainder of this report as the SHAD I study, were complex, but did not show clear relationships between participation in the SHAD tests and adverse long-term health effects. Questions about the SHAD I study from veterans and from Congressmen Mike Thompson and Dennis Rehberg about certain aspects of the study resulted in the IOM conducting some additional analyses and preparing a short follow-up publication in 2008 (IOM, 2008).

The SHAD I study examined both the mortality experience of SHAD veterans and the health status of the surviving veterans. Data on health status were collected through a survey of the members of the study population who were assumed to be alive at the time of the study. Responses were received from 61 percent of the SHAD veterans and 47 percent of the comparison population surviving at the time of the study. The modest size of the study population and the level of response to the survey meant that the findings in the SHAD I study could not be considered conclusive because uncommon or subtle health effects would be difficult to discern. Furthermore, the SHAD I study had little basis for assessing the potential impact of differences among SHAD veterans in their levels of possible exposure to the agents used in the tests.

Continuing concerns about potential health effects from exposures during SHAD testing and an interest in further evaluation of the health of this population led to a request in the Caregivers and Veterans Omnibus Health Services Act of 2010 (PL 111-163) for an expanded IOM study of the SHAD test participant and comparison populations. This study, carried out by the Committee on Shipboard Hazard and Defense (SHAD) II between June 2011 and October 2015 is the subject of this report. The new study expanded on the previous IOM work by making use of additional years of health care experience, including an analysis of data from Medicare, which captures most health care encounters for people who have attained the age of 65.[1]

In finding no overall differences in all-cause mortality between SHAD participants and comparison groups, the SHAD II analysis agreed with the results of the previous IOM study. However, it differed in that, with an additional 7 years of follow up, it did not find an elevation in heart disease mortality except in one of the exposure groups examined. The SHAD II analysis found no clear differences in degree of illness between SHAD participants and the comparison group. This result was consistent with the absence of differences in self-reported hospitalizations noted in SHAD I, but not in accord with the SHAD I survey responses that indicated overall worse health among SHAD veterans.

This report provides background on Project SHAD testing, describes the study population and the health outcomes data used in the new analysis, and presents the findings of the analysis.

## STUDY CHARGE AND COMMITTEE ACTIVITIES

The IOM Committee on Shipboard Hazard and Defense (SHAD) II was charged with conducting a new epidemiological study of the potential long-term health effects of participation in the SHAD testing. The study charge appears in Box 1-1.

In carrying out its work, the committee held five in-person meetings and numerous meetings via conference call. Two meetings included public sessions at which SHAD veterans described to the committee their experiences during the tests and responded to questions. Panels represented veterans from several specific tests, and a group of veterans who had served as part of the Project SHAD Technical Staff (PSTS) also shared some of their experiences and perspectives with the IOM committee. Agendas listing the participants in these meetings can be found in Appendix B. Additional discussion of the input provided at these meetings appears in Chapter 2.

The committee oversaw a search of the scientific literature to identify reports published in 2000 or later that might update information on the potential health effects from exposure to the agents, simulants, decontaminants, and tracers[2] used in the tests. Committee members also discussed findings from their review of the redacted technical reports describing the tests and planned elements of study design.

---

[1] As of December 31, 2011, the end of the follow-up period for this study, 83 percent of SHAD test participants assumed alive were 65 years of age or older.

[2] The literature review included all of the substances reported to have been used in the tests to allow for the possibility that substances previously thought to be harmless (e.g., simulants and tracers) may subsequently have been found to have health risks.

## APPROACH TO THE STUDY

The committee's interest was in evaluating whether the long-term health of SHAD veterans has been adversely affected by their exposures during SHAD testing. The committee uses "long-term" to mean persisting or recurring conditions as well as those appearing several years or more after exposure. The committee evaluated the causes of SHAD veterans' deaths since the 1960s and the diagnoses assigned at hospital and outpatient visits in data from the VA health system and from Medicare from 1999 through 2011. The analysis included two approaches. One focused on testing hypotheses about specific exposures and health outcomes that the committee concluded were suggested by a review of the scientific literature. The other exploratory approach was based on testing the more general hypothesis that the health or mortality experience of the population of SHAD veterans (or certain subgroups) differed from that of the veterans in the comparison population.

Specifically, the committee sought to address the following questions:

Research Question 1: Is participation in SHAD tests that used certain agents, simulants, tracers, or decontaminants associated with differences in long-term health effects?

> *Objective 1*: Test the hypotheses that exposure to specific agents is associated with greater incidence of specific health effects (e.g., *Coxiella burnetii* and endocarditis; sarin and neurological effects).
>
> *Objective 2*: Test the hypotheses that exposure to specific agents is associated with greater mortality from specific causes (e.g., *C. burnetii* and endocarditis; betapropiolactone and cancers).

Research Question 2: How does the health of Project SHAD participants compare with that of a comparison population of veterans who served on similar ships or in similar units that did not participate in the SHAD tests?

> *Objective 1*: Compare, as appropriate, the cumulative incidence or prevalence of specified chronic conditions and cancers between participants and controls using VA and Centers for Medicare & Medicaid Services inpatient and outpatient data
>
> *Objective 2*: Compare the mortality experience of participant and control populations using vital status information from VA, the National Death Index, and state vital records offices.

The SHAD testing involved use of active chemical and biological agents, simulants, tracers, and decontaminants (see Box 1-2).[3] Active chemical and biological agents were potential weapons and known to be debilitating or even fatal in the short term. Simulants were substances that shared certain chemical or biological characteristics of the active agents but were considered at the time to be relatively safe to use. For example, *Bacillus globigii* (BG) has been used for

---

[3] The following substances were included in the SHAD I review but were not included in the update of literature for this study: bis-hydrogen phosphite and phosphorus-32. These tracers were disseminated with VX over a barge in the Flower Drum II test. No personnel have been identified as participants in this test.

**BOX 1-2**
**Agents, Simulants, Tracers, and Decontaminants Reported by DoD to Be Used in SHAD Testing**

**Active Agents**

**Biological**

*Coxiella burnetii*
*Pasteurella tularensis (Francisella tularensis)*
Staphylococcal enterotoxin type B, or SEB

**Chemical**

Sarin
VX

**Simulants**

**Biological**

*Bacillus globigii* or BG
*Escherichia coli or E. coli*
*Serratia marcescens* or SM

**Chemicalaa**

Diethylphthlate
Methyl acetoacetate or MAA
Sulfur dioxide
Trioctyl phosphate, or (tris(2-ethylhexyl) phosphate) or TOF or TEHP

**Tracers**

Calcofluor
Diethylphthlate mixed with 0.1 percent of fluorescent dye DF-504
Uranine or sodium flourescein
Zinc cadmium sulfide

**Decontaminants**

Betapropiolactone
Calcium hypochlorite

many years as a simulant for the aerosol behavior of the active biological agent *Bacillus anthracis*, which causes the disease anthrax. Tracers were substances used to track the movement of test agents or simulants.

To test the hypotheses generated by a review of published literature (Research Question 1), the committee looked at those SHAD participants with exposure to particular agents and compared their experience of specific health effects with the unexposed comparison group. For its broader analysis (Research Question 2), the committee compared health outcomes in the participant group with those of service members from similar vessels and units. Additional analyses considered the potential effects of differences in exposures to types of agents (e.g., any biological agent, any chemical agent) and in numbers of exposures based on numbers of tests and trials within tests.

The comparison population was made up of the crews of Navy vessels identified to be as similar as possible to those participating in the Project SHAD tests. Similarly, the comparison population of Marines was men in units comparable to those that participated in the SHAD tests. Identification of the comparison ships and Marine units is described in greater detail in Chapters 2 and 3. All of the study participants and comparison population were men.

## CHALLENGES FOR THE STUDY

Several of the challenges involved in carrying out this study are typical of studies to examine the potential health effects from past occupational exposures. For example, the SHAD tests took place in the 1960s and were not intended to study the health of the participants. However, occupational health researchers often have to turn to decades-old records that may be incomplete and are not designed for use in estimating a workplace exposure. Other challenges are specific to the unusual circumstances of the Project SHAD testing.

The committee reviewed the information available from both DoD fact sheets and the publicly available portions of the reports written for each of the 21 SHAD tests. All of the study participants had in common their participation in at least one of the Project SHAD test trials, but it became clear to the committee that several subgroups could be defined on the basis of the particular agents, simulants, tracers, or decontaminants that had been used in the specific tests. One subgroup of particular interest was the crews of five light tug boats that had a role in the only SHAD tests reported to have used active biological warfare agents in addition to the simulants used in many of the other tests. Rosters for the crews of these small vessels were not archived as crew rosters were for most Navy ships. Although the tugs participated in six tests, crew members have been identified as a group in conjunction with only one test in January 1965. Moreover, it was not possible to identify comparable ships that could contribute crew members to the comparison population. Identification of members of the PSTS was also limited to a single document from January 1965.

The men who served on the USS *George Eastman* were also of special interest because this test ship was the only manned vessel reported to be involved in trials using active chemical warfare agents in addition to simulants. Focused analysis for each of these subgroups was a challenge because of the relatively small numbers of people involved in each group. Chapter 3 discusses analytical issues further.

Ideally, studies to assess whether environmental or occupational exposures are associated with adverse health effects are able to incorporate quantitative information about the amount of exposure each member of the study population received. The concentration of a substance in each subject's blood or urine might be used, for example. Often, however, studies must rely on indirect indicators of exposure such as the concentration of a substance in the air where a subject worked and the amount of time (e.g., days, months, years) the subject worked there. For this study, the committee's assessment of the exposures received by participants in the SHAD tests was constrained by the limits of the available documentation. Information on the concentrations of test agents, simulants, tracers, and decontaminants used in the tests largely remains classified. To the committee's knowledge, no biological samples were collected from the participants that could be used to measure individuals' internal dose of specific substances used in the tests. In a few tests, contact with these substances was assessed using mouth washes, nasal swabs, or clothing patches. For two tests, such information was available in a qualitative form (e.g., high, medium, low exposure) that was not sufficient to aid the analysis. Although the SHAD tests generally used air samplers placed in various locations of a ship to measure the presence and concentration of a test substance, the data that were collected are among those that remain classified. Moreover, no information was available to show the location of individual crew members during a test, making the sampler data unhelpful in confidently distinguishing potential exposure levels among crew members.

The IOM requested declassification of additional material pertaining to the tests and exposures, including data on particle size, air sampler locations and sampler results, and movie films of some of the tests. A preliminary DoD review resulted in the conclusion that additional material for only one test was appropriate for declassification. Material on the other tests was not considered suitable for declassification because of its potential to reveal ship vulnerabilities to chemical or biological agents. At the time this report was written, no additional materials had been declassified and provided to the committee.

## TOPICS BEYOND THE SCOPE OF THE STUDY

Some topics were considered beyond the scope of the study. For the SHAD I study, the IOM staff made a detailed review of Navy quarterly unit rosters and daily personnel diaries and of Marine Corps monthly personnel rosters and company diaries as part of a validation of the study participants identified by DoD as being present during the time of the SHAD tests. In that review of archival materials, the IOM identified several additional likely SHAD test participants and provided these names to DoD to augment its database. Since that time and as described by Government Accountability Office (GAO) reports (2004, 2008), contractors working on behalf of DoD have continued searching records to identify veterans potentially involved in Project SHAD and other chemical and biological warfare testing.

Consistent with the charge for the current study to use the same population of test participants and the same comparison population as in the first study, the IOM did not repeat its independent review of personnel diaries and quarterly reports. However, the IOM did receive an updated listing of SHAD participants from DoD, in order to use the most recent roster of participants. Thus, the analysis for the current report included any additional test participants who had been identified in the years since the first IOM study was concluded. As described in Chapter 3, nine additional test participants were identified through this update.

Several veterans who had served as members of the PSTS reported that they had been administered vaccines against certain biological warfare agents such as those that cause tularemia (*P/F tularensis*) and Q fever (*C. burnetii*). They noted that the vaccinations had been recorded on lists that did not become part of their permanent medical records or personnel folders. Because information linking specific vaccinations to specific individuals was not available, the committee could not include the vaccinations as separate exposure factors in the study. However, and as noted in the data and methods chapter, the tug and PSTS group was considered to have several unique exposures that should be taken into account in their analysis as a special subgroup.

Several SHAD veterans have also expressed concerns about the potential for exposure to radiation from their service because two of the ships used in SHAD had also been used to monitor nuclear tests conducted in the Pacific Ocean in the 1950s (Naval History and Heritage Command, 2015a,b). The two ships were the USS *George Eastman*, which served as a target vessel in six SHAD tests, and the USS *Granville S. Hall,* which served as a laboratory ship for many SHAD tests.[4] In addition, tug crews who participated in the 1965 SHAD test Shady Grove spent some time on Johnston Atoll, which had been used for nuclear testing in 1962 (Personal communication, J. Alderson, U.S. Navy Reserve (Ret.), January 22, 2013). Radiation was not specifically a SHAD-related exposure, but various factors noted in Chapter 3 resulted in these groups receiving special analytical consideration.

As has been noted, Project SHAD was part of a larger testing program designated Project 112. Because the charge to the committee was to study SHAD exposures and use the same participant and comparison populations as in the previous IOM study, the committee did not attempt to include participants in the other Project 112 tests that took place between December 1962 and May 1974 (see DoD, 2015).

Veterans and others have raised questions about the ethics and legality of the SHAD testing (described further in Chapter 2). While many issues attend consideration of Project SHAD, this committee was not charged with reviewing the merits of the program. The focus was on the scientific question of whether test participation is associated with adverse long-term health effects.

## THE COMMITTEE'S REPORT

This report reviews the information available on the individual Project SHAD tests and the agents, simulants, tracers, and decontaminants used in them for an analysis of the association between participation in the tests or specific exposures in the tests and long-term health effects. Specifically, Chapter 2 provides background on the SHAD tests, previous studies of SHAD veterans, and some of the concerns and input SHAD veterans shared with the committee in its public workshops. Chapter 3 describes the rationale for the committee's approach to and design for the study. Chapter 4 presents results of the analysis of the mortality data, and Chapter 5 focuses on the analysis of morbidity data. Chapter 6 provides a discussion of the findings from the analysis and their implications, and notes the strengths and weaknesses of the study. Included as appendixes are biographical sketches of committee members (Appendix A), agendas for the committee's public sessions (Appendix B), information from the review of recent literature on each of the test substances (Appendix C), additional information on data and methods used for analysis (Appendix D), units participating in Project SHAD tests and units selected as comparisons (Appendix E), and diagnostic codes used to define health outcomes (Appendix F).

## REFERENCES

DoD (Department of Defense). 2015. *Project 112/SHAD fact sheets.* http://www.health.mil/Military-Health-Topics/Health-Readiness/Environmental-Exposures/Project-112-SHAD/Fact-Sheets (accessed October 1, 2015).

GAO (General Accounting Office). 2004. *Chemical and biological defense: DoD needs to continue to collect and provide information on tests and potentially exposed personnel.* GAO-04-410. Washington, DC: General Accounting Office.

---

[4] There was an anecdotal report that at least one ship set off a radiation alarm in a Hawaiian harbor (Morris, 2004, Tab 6).

GAO (Government Accountability Office). 2008. *Chemical and biological defense: DoD and VA need to improve efforts to identify and notify individuals potentially exposed during chemical and biological tests.* GAO-08-366. Washington, DC: Government Accountability Office.

IOM (Institute of Medicine). 2007. *Long-term health effects of participation in Project SHAD (Shipboard Hazard and Defense).* Washington, DC: The National Academies Press.

IOM. 2008. *Response to 15 February 2008 letter from Congressmen Mike Thompson and Dennis Rehberg.* Letter from Frederick J. Erdtmann, Director, Medical Follow-up Agency, Institute of Medicine. http://iom.nationalacademies.org/~/media/Files/Report%20Files/2007/Long-Term-Health-Effects-of-Participation-in-Project-SHAD-Shipboard-Hazard-and-Defense/SHAD%20Response%20Letter.pdf (accessed January 7, 2014).

Morris, D. D. 2004. *The Department of Defense identification of participants and exposures in Projects 112 and Shipboard Hazard and Defense.* M.P.H. thesis, Morris, Dee Dodson: George Washington University.

Naval History and Heritage Command. 2015a. *George Eastman.* http://www.history.navy.mil/research/histories/ship-histories/danfs/g/george-eastman.html (accessed October 15, 2015).

Naval History and Heritage Command. 2015b. *Granville S. Hall (YAG-40).* http://www.history.navy.mil/research/histories/ship-histories/danfs/g/granville-s-hall-yag-40.html (accessed October 15, 2015).

# 2

# Background

The central task of the committee was to carry out an epidemiologic analysis of potential associations between Project Shipboard Hazard and Defense (SHAD) test exposures and long-term health outcomes. An understanding of the background to the tests and the details of how they were carried out informed the committee's approach to the study and provides context for the concerns and perspectives of the veterans who participated in these tests.

This chapter reviews the history of Project SHAD and efforts to reconstruct information about the tests and identify military service members who participated in them. It presents summary information about the tests and discusses a few in greater detail to illustrate some of the variation among them. It provides a brief review of studies of the health of SHAD veterans, including the design and findings of SHAD I, the previous Institute of Medicine (IOM) study of the long-term health effects of associated with participation in Project SHAD (IOM, 2007). Finally, this chapter describes the concerns of the veterans who were assigned to the ships and other units that participated in the tests.

## PROJECT SHAD[1]

### Origins and Termination

During the Cold War, the U.S. government was concerned not only about nuclear threats from the Soviet Union and China but also that the Soviet Union had programs to develop biological and chemical warfare agents and delivery systems. At the start of the Kennedy administration in 1961, Secretary of Defense Robert McNamara requested a broad assessment of the military challenges facing the United States and military readiness to meet these challenges. Among the approximately 150 numbered projects that resulted, Project 112 addressed biological and chemical warfare capabilities and defense (DoD, 2003c).

[1] The description in this report of the history of Project SHAD and the efforts by DoD since 2000 to provide documentation of test activities draws extensively from two unpublished documents. One document is a report submitted to Congress in 2003 by Assistant Secretary of Defense for Health Affairs William Winkenwerder. The other source is a master's thesis prepared by Dee Morris, who led DoD work to assemble information for the Project 112 and Project SHAD fact sheets and to compile additional information about the tests for the SHAD I study by the Institute of Medicine.

In 1962, when Project 112 began, the effects of varying climates and terrain on potential biological and chemical weapons were not known, nor was the feasibility and effectiveness of decontamination in varying settings and environments. The classified testing conducted for Project 112 was designed to improve knowledge in these areas, and some of the tests—those now referred to as the Project SHAD component of Project 112—focused on ships and the marine environment (Morris, 2004).

The testing program was managed by the Deseret Test Center (DTC), which was established by the U.S. Army in June 1962 at Fort Douglas, Utah. DTC was funded and staffed by all of the military services. The services submitted testing requirements annually, and test objectives and priorities were determined at joint planning conferences by service and joint and combatant command representatives (DoD, 2003c; GAO, 2004). Initial plans for Project 112 called for tests to take place "in the Pacific Ocean or on land in Alaska, Hawaii, and the then-Panama Canal Zone" (DoD, 2003c, unnumbered p. 5). Ultimately, some additional locations were also used. It is evident from the test plans and descriptions that the tests were intended to evaluate operational characteristics of ships and protective and dissemination equipment as well as the behavior of the test agents in marine environments; these tests were clearly not concerned with assessing health impacts. A modern analogy is the testing for the integrity of important buildings in the face of Homeland Security concerns. Tests to evaluate the effects of the agents on human health would have required different designs.

According to the Department of Defense (DoD), 134 classified tests were planned for land or sea, involving open-air use of various combinations of active agents (both chemical and biological), simulants, tracers, and decontaminants (DoD, 2003c). Of the planned Project 112 tests, 50 were completed and 84 were cancelled (DoD, 2015). The completed tests included 21[2] that involved Navy vessels and that DoD designated as SHAD tests (DoD, 2014) in its 2000-2003 review and declassification of materials related to the testing program. Each SHAD test was conducted over a period of weeks or months and included several "trials," each of which was typically conducted on a separate day. Table 2-1 provides a list of the designations and features of the SHAD tests. The first SHAD test began in January of 1963, and the final SHAD test using active agents or simulants was conducted in 1969. Some Project 112 testing continued in the period 1970-1974, all of it conducted at Dugway Proving Ground, Utah.

DoD has cited several developments as contributing to the termination of Project 112 and Project SHAD (DoD, 2003c). In November 1969, President Nixon announced a moratorium on biological weapons testing and that research on biological weapons should focus on defense, including "on techniques of immunization, and on measures of controlling and preventing the spread of disease" (Nixon, 1969).[3] Funding for DTC was "severely curtailed" by mid-1971, and the center was closed in 1973 (DoD, 2003c, unnumbered p. 7). Upon its closure, most of its records were transferred to Dugway Proving Ground (Morris, 2004, p. 6).

---

[2] Of 21 tests designated as SHAD tests by DoD, 20 involved potential exposure to agents, simulants, tracers, or decontaminants. Test DTC 70-C, which took place in 1972 and 1973 (DoD, 2003b), involved only passive air sampling to characterize naturally occurring airborne particles in the marine atmosphere.

[3] Also in November 1969, PL 91-121 (50 U.S.C. 1512) required a determination by the Secretary of Defense that transport or testing of any chemical or biological warfare agents in the United States was in the interest of national security and that any precautionary measures recommended by the Secretary of Health, Education, and Welfare first be implemented. In 1970, the Clean Air Act (PL 91-604) authorized the development of federal and state regulations to limit the release of harmful substances into the air (see EPA, 2014).

**TABLE 2-1** Features of Shipboard Hazard and Defense (SHAD) Tests, 1963 to 1969

| Test | Date | No. of Trials | Location | Participating Units (# trials) | Agent or Simulant Used[a] | Protective Gear/ Decontamination | Purpose |
|---|---|---|---|---|---|---|---|
| Eager Belle I (Test 63-1) | Jan, Mar 1963 | 19 | Pacific Ocean, west of Oahu, Hawaii | USS *George Eastman* | *Bacillus globigii* (BG) | | Test effectiveness of face masks and protective devices for ship |
| Eager Belle II (Test 63-1) | Feb, Mar, Jun 1963 | 14 | Pacific Ocean, west of Oahu | USS *George Eastman* (11)<br>USS *Carpenter* (1)<br>USS *Navarro* (1)<br>USS *Tioga County* (1)<br>USMC Medium Helicopter Squadron 161 | *Bacillus globigii* (BG) | | Obtain information (1) on models for travel of biological aerosols; (2) on weapon system performance; (3) for design of future tests |
| Autumn Gold (Test 63-2) | May 1963 | 9 | 60 miles west-southwest of Oahu | USS *Carpenter* (9)<br>USS *Hoel* (7)<br>USS *Navarro* (9)<br>USS *Tioga County* (9)<br>Marine Air Group 13 | *Bacillus globigii* (BG) | M17 and Mark V masks | Test aerosol penetration of ships under three readiness conditions; estimate magnitude and persistence of dispersed agent after washdown; evaluate masks |
| Errand Boy (Test 64-1) | Sep 1963 | 8 | East Loch, Pearl Harbor, Hawaii | USS *George Eastman* | *Bacillus globigii* (BG) | Betapropiolactone (BPL) | Test decontamination procedures for external surfaces |
| Flower Drum I (Test 64-2) | Feb-Apr, Aug-Sept 1964 | 31 | Pacific Ocean, off coast of Hawaii | USS *George Eastman* | Sarin (GB)<br>Methyl acetoacetate (MAA)<br>Sulfur dioxide (SO2) | M5 Protective Ensemble for disseminator crew Others wore MK5, M7A1 and M17 masks inside the Safety Citadel | Find simulant for GB, assess penetration of vapor of GB and simulant |
| Shady Grove (Test 64-4) | May 1964; Jan-Apr 1965 | 25 | Pacific Ocean | 5 Army tugs<br>Marine Air Group 13<br><br>USN Patrol Squadrons 4 and 6<br>USN | *Coxiella burnetii* (OU)<br>*Pasteurella tularensis* (UL)<br>*Bacillus globigii* (BG) | | Determine infectivity, viability, and atmospheric diffusion of UL; assess capability of weapon system; evaluate procedures for tests with pathogenic |

| Test | Date | No. of Trials | Location | Participating Units (# trials) | Agent or Simulant Used[a] | Protective Gear/ Decontamination | Purpose |
|---|---|---|---|---|---|---|---|
| | | | | AEWBARONPAC | Zinc cadmium sulfide (tracer) | | agents |
| Flower Drum II (Test 64-2) | Nov-Dec 1964 | 10 | Pacific Ocean, off the coast of Oahu | USN tug ATF 105<br>Unmanned USN barge YFN-811 | VX<br>Phosphorous 32<br>Bis (2 ethyl-hexyl) hydrogen | Shipboard water washdown | Test effectiveness of shipboard water washdown against VX; obtain operational experience for planning test designated Fearless Johnny |
| Copper Head (Test 65-1) | Jan-Feb 1965 | 10 | Atlantic Ocean, off the coast of Newfound-land, Canada | USS *Power* | *Bacillus globigii* (BG)<br>Zinc cadmium sulfide (FP) | Betapropiolactone (BPL) | Test in a frigid marine environment: extent of aerosol penetration into an operational ship under three conditions of readiness; compare travel of a biological cloud with diffusion model predictions; effectiveness of BPL; operational feasibility of deck washdown system; performance of spray tank system |
| High Low (Test 65-13) | Jan-Feb 1965 | 33 | Pacific Ocean, off the coast of San Diego | USS *Berkeley*<br>USS *Fechteler*<br>USS *Okanogan*<br>USS *Wexford County* | Methyl acetoacetate (MAA) | Protective masks | Using a simulant, investigate the potential penetration of a cloud of sarin into four types of naval ships |
| Big Tom (Test 65-6) | Apr-Jun 1965 | 19 | Off the coast of Oahu, and on Oahu | USS *Carbonero* | *Bacillus globigii* (BG)<br><br>Fluorescent particles of zinc cadmium sulfide (tracers) | Betapropiolactone (BPL) (USS *Carbonero*) | Evaluate the feasibility of a biological attack on an island complex; evaluate doctrine and tactics for such an attack |

| Test | Date | No. of Trials | Location | Participating Units (# trials) | Agent or Simulant Used[a] | Protective Gear/ Decontamination | Purpose |
|---|---|---|---|---|---|---|---|
| Magic Sword (Test 65-4) | May 1965 | 8 | Pacific Ocean, off the coast of Baker Island (and on Baker Island)[b] | USS *George Eastman* | Uninfected mosquitoes | Nonpersistent insecticide<br>Heat<br><br>(DDT on Baker Island) | Study the (1) feasibility of offshore release of *Aedes aegypti* mosquitoes, (2) mosquito biting habits, (3) trap technology, and (4) delivery of mosquitoes to remote sites |
| Fearless Johnny (Test 65-17) | Aug-Sep 1965 | 17 | Pacific Ocean, southwest of Oahu | USS *George Eastman*<br>2 light tugs[c]<br>USN Patrol Squadron 6 (Naval aviation unit) | VX (3 trials)<br>Diethylphthalate (DEP) with dye (14 trials) | Water washdown system | Evaluate contamination (external, internal) from aerial dissemination of nerve agent simulant; test effectiveness of decontamination process; assess impact of gross VX contamination |
| Purple Sage (Test 66-5) | Jan-Feb 1966 | 21 | Pacific Ocean, off the coast of San Diego | USS *Herbert J. Thomas* | Methyl acetoacetate (MAA) | Protective mask (MK5 or M17) | Evaluate the effectiveness of the Shipboard Toxicological Operational Protection System (STOPS) against gaseous chemical warfare agents; evaluate the impact of protective masks on crew efficiency |
| Scarlet Sage (Test 66-6) | Feb-Mar 1966 | 19 | Pacific Ocean, off the coast of San Diego | USS *Herbert J. Thomas*<br>AVR boat *North Island* | *Bacillus globigii* (BG) | Water washdown | Evaluate the effectiveness of the Shipboard Toxicological Operational Protective System (STOPS) against a biological aerosol; determine level of contamination and effectiveness of decontamination system; evaluate nasal-pharyngeal wash for detecting inhalation of biological aerosol |

| Test | Date | No. of Trials | Location | Participating Units (# trials) | Agent or Simulant Used[a] | Protective Gear/ Decontamination | Purpose |
|---|---|---|---|---|---|---|---|
| Half Note (Test 66-13) | Aug-Sep 1966 | ≥27 | Pacific Ocean, south-southwest of Oahu | USS *George Eastman*<br>5 Army tugs<br>USS *Carbonero* (BG release) | *Escherichia coli* (EC)<br>*Serratia marcescens* (SM)<br>*Bacillus globigii* (BG)<br>Calcofluor (tracers)<br>Zinc cadmium sulfide | Calcium hypochlorite in water (USS *Carbonero*) | Determine decay rates of nonpathogenic organisms in marine environment<br>Assess contamination hazards for USS *Carbonero* |
| Folded Arrow (Test 68-71) | Apr-May 1968 | 11 | Pacific Ocean, south-southwest of Oahu and off the coast of Oahu | 5 Army tugs<br>USS *Carbonero* (disseminator) | *Bacillus globigii* (BG) | Betapropiolactone (BPL)<br>Calcium hypochlorite | Study over-ocean downwind travel of biological aerosols; demonstrate capability of submarine weapon system for biological attack against islands and ports; Evaluate contamination hazard to submarine crew |
| Test 69-31 | Aug-Sep 1968 | 16 | Off the coast of San Diego | USS *Herbert J. Thomas* | Methyl acetoacetate (MAA)<br>*Bacillus globigii* (BG) | | Evaluate the continued effectiveness of STOPS after operational deployment |
| Speckled Start (Test 68-50) | Sep-Oct 1968 | 21 | Pacific Ocean, Eniwetok Atoll | 5 Army tugs<br>USAF 4533rd Tactical Test Squadron, 33rd Tactical Fighter Wing | Staphylococcus enterotoxin B (SEB)<br>*Bacillus globigii* (BG, dry)<br>Uranine dye | | Determine the potential casualty area and associated casualty levels for aerosols dispersed by the F-4/AB45Y-4/PG2 weapon system |
| Test 69-32 | Apr-Jun 1969 | 27 | Pacific Ocean, southwest of Hawaii | 5 Army tugs<br>USN A-4C aircraft from VC-1 squadron | *Escherichia coli* (EC) (13 trials)<br>*Serratia marcescens* (SM) (14 trials)<br>*Bacillus globigii* (BG)<br>Calcofluor (tracer) | | Evaluate the effect of sunlight on the viability of biological aerosols disseminated in a temperate environment at about sunrise and sunset |

| Test | Date | No. of Trials | Location | Participating Units (# trials) | Agent or Simulant Used[a] | Protective Gear/ Decontamination | Purpose |
|---|---|---|---|---|---|---|---|
| Test 69-10 | May 1969 | ≥4 | Vieques Island, Puerto Rico | USS *Fort Snelling* (LSD-30)<br>USMC Landing Force Carib 1-69/BLT 1/8 (2nd Marine Division)<br>USMC VMA-324, MAG-32 | Trioctyl phosphate (TOF) (also known as tri(2-ethylhexyl) phosphate [TEHP]) | | Determine the operational effects during an amphibious landing of a persistent chemical agent spray attack on troops wearing protective clothing and on contamination of troops, ships, and equipment |

NOTES: The USS *Granville S. Hall* was present during the following SHAD tests as an escort ship or to provide laboratory facilities for analysis of samples collected during SHAD tests: Eager Belle II, Autumn Gold, Flower Drum I, Shady Grove, Big Tom, Fearless Johnny, Folded Arrow, Half Note, Speckled Start, and Test 69-32. It did not serve as a test ship during SHAD tests. Test 70-C did not involve the release of a test agent or use of tracers or decontaminants. It is not included here and was not included in any of the analyses discussed in this report. AEWBARONPAC = Airborne Early Warning Barrier Squadron Pacific; MAG = Marine Air Group; USAF = United States Air Force; USMC = United States Marine Corps; USN = United States Navy

[a] Active agents are listed first, followed by simulants and tracers.

[b] The portion of the test conducted on Baker Island has not been included in any of the analyses discussed in this report.

[c] Two light tugs were reported to serve as couriers (not test vessels) during Fearless Johnny.

## Reconstruction of Information About Project SHAD

During the 1990s, some veterans raised concerns to the Department of Veterans Affairs (VA) that they had health problems that were the result of exposures during the Project 112 and Project SHAD tests. Because the testing programs were classified, service members reported that they were forbidden to discuss their participation the tests (e.g., Personal communication, G. Arnold, SHAD veteran, USS *Navarro*, February 23, 2012),[4] and VA had little information about the tests. Congressional inquiries on behalf of SHAD veterans received varying responses from the Department of the Army, which serves as DoD's executive agent for chemical and biological testing. At least one response from the Department of the Army noted the existence of some of the tests and that veterans who felt they might have service-connected health problems could submit claims to VA, and the Army would respond to VA requests for information (Beard, 1996).

In May 2000, a series of investigative television news reports brought public attention to the SHAD testing.[5] In August 2000, the acting secretary of VA, Hershel Gober, sent a request to DoD for information about Project SHAD testing, including lists of the names and dates of tests, the agents used, and the military units and individuals who were participants in the tests (Gober, 2000). DoD's efforts to prepare this material required locating information contained primarily in paper records of classified activities that had occurred 30 to 40 years earlier. By October 2003, DoD had produced a list of the Project 112 and Project SHAD tests that are known to have been planned, and it prepared unclassified fact sheets about each test that was conducted (see DoD, 2015).

Within DoD, responsibility to assemble the information requested by VA was eventually assigned to the Office of the Special Assistant to the Secretary of Defense for Gulf War Illnesses, Medical Readiness, and Military Deployments.[6] Their investigation into SHAD testing included a review of files by the Army, requests for additional information from other military commands or units likely to have received copies of the reports, and interviews with people with information about the SHAD testing program. It also resulted in interagency meetings that included representatives of VA, DoD, and the Department of Health and Human Services (HHS). An unpublished paper by the DoD staff member assigned to lead this work provides insight into the challenges of locating records of the SHAD test program and reconstructing the program's history (Morris, 2004).

The first phase of the investigation focused on gathering information about the SHAD tests designated Autumn Gold, Shady Grove, and Copper Head. The first two of these tests were identified by the acting VA Secretary Gober and by Congressman Mike Thompson (California) as being of interest, and the Army had reported in its initial response to VA that it had

[4] In 2011, DoD issued a memorandum that released veterans from any nondisclosure obligations (including any "secrecy oaths") related to their potential exposure to chemical or biological agents (DoD, 2011). This release allows for discussions of health concerns, but it does not authorize release of technical or operational information. No written secrecy oaths related to the Project SHAD tests were located by DoD during its investigation into the Project 112 testing (Personal communication, Michael E. Kilpatrick, Force Health Protection and Readiness Programs, Department of Defense, to the IOM Committee on Shipboard Hazard and Defense II, January 19, 2012).

[5] The series of reports were presented by Vince Gonzales on *CBS News* (Murphy, 2003), based on investigations by Eric Longabardi.

[6] This organization is now known as the Office of the Deputy Assistant Secretary of Defense for Health Readiness Policy and Oversight.

unclassified information on Copper Head (Morris, 2004). The second phase of the investigation was to cover the remaining SHAD tests as time and resources permitted, with priority given to any tests named in claims that veterans had filed with VA (Morris, 2004). The investigation into SHAD tests also led to the identification and documentation of land-based tests that were part of the broader Project 112 testing program.

Obtaining information about SHAD tests was challenging because the term "Project SHAD" was not in wide use (e.g., in test plans or reports) at the time the tests were conducted and so was not a useful search term in databases (Morris, 2004, p. 8). The investigation began with a search by the staff at Dugway Proving Ground of classified technical holdings there. The Dugway staff identified 38 classified documents relevant to Project SHAD, and copies were sent to the investigators, who reviewed them for "medically relevant information" (described as "i.e. where, when, to what vessel/unit"). Later in the process, the SHAD investigators made a further on-site search of the materials held at Dugway, which resulted in finding additional documents as well as films of some of the tests.[7] Some documents related to the tests had originally been distributed beyond DTC and were located by the investigators in files at the U.S. Army Edgewood Chemical Biological Center (Edgewood, Maryland) and the Naval Surface Warfare Center (Dahlgren, Virginia). Documents were also identified and obtained through the catalogue and collection of the Defense Technical Information Center (DTIC). In addition, the investigators also conferred with J. Clifton Spendlove, the technical director for the tests, about the testing program and the documents and films found.

The SHAD investigators requested declassification of documents by the appropriate originating agencies in the Army and the Navy (Morris, 2004), but the volume of material (more than 28,000 pages) could not be reviewed in a timely manner by those agencies. Plans to seek declassification of entire documents were abandoned, and as of 2004, approximately 400 pages had been declassified after 14 separate requests (Morris, 2004).

Investigators used clues in the classified documents to guide them to unclassified operational and personnel records at the National Archives and Records Administration (NARA) in College Park, Maryland. VA agreed to accept a record of an individual's assignment to a participating unit or vessel at the time of a SHAD test as sufficient evidence of participation in the test. To compile rosters of personnel qualifying as SHAD test participants, DoD investigators examined quarterly personnel summaries for the periods immediately before and after SHAD test dates (Morris, 2004). Personnel who were named on both summaries were presumed to have been test participants. If a person's name appeared on only one summary, daily muster rolls had to be checked to clarify whether he should be considered a test participant. As of 2003, DoD had identified approximately 5,900 individuals who were assigned to ships or other military units that participated in SHAD or other Project 112 tests (GAO, 2004).

A 2004 review by the General Accounting Office (GAO) described DoD's processes for finding materials to identify Project 112 tests as satisfactory: "It appears that DOD used a reasonable approach for identifying the locations of records and source documents, particularly since some of the Project 112 tests were conducted more than 40 years ago and the record-keeping systems were much less sophisticated than today's" (GAO, 2004, p. 11). The GAO review included examination of materials that DoD investigators had used (including selective examination of materials stored at Dugway Proving Ground) and interviews with staff members at DoD and former officials and managers from DTC. However, GAO (2004, 2008) also

[7] Morris (2004) reports that some of the films were transferred to other formats but that sound tracks were lost. The committee requested copies of this video material, but DoD declined to publicly release it.

concluded that further DoD effort would be warranted to identify additional military and civilian personnel who may have been participants in SHAD or other Project 112 tests.[8]

Some of the SHAD veterans who presented written or oral statements to this committee (e.g., February 2012 IOM meeting; Personal communication, J. Alderson, U.S. Navy Reserve (Ret.), January 22, 2013) expressed views skeptical of the thoroughness of the DoD investigation and that additional information about the tests is available. The committee's understanding is that additional, and potentially relevant, material on SHAD tests exists and remains classified. The IOM committee requested declassification of 21 additional elements from at least nine documents from DoD in August 2012. In January 2014, an additional request was made for release of multiple films made of Project SHAD tests. None of the requested materials were cleared for public release as of this writing.

## THE SHAD TESTS

Figure 2-1 shows the timing of tests that DoD has identified as being part of Project SHAD. Table 2-1 includes information about when and where the tests were conducted, the military units that participated, and the substances used. Additional description of each of the tests is provided in the annex to this chapter. Two of the tests have been excluded from most of the subsequent discussion and analysis in this report because no participants in the tests have been identified (Flower Drum II), or because the test did not involve the release of any substances (DTC 70-C).

As Table 2-1 illustrates, the SHAD tests had varying goals and test conditions. Some tests used only simulants, and others used active biological or chemical agents. The tests also differed in that some were carried out with "regular" Navy ships and crews, while others used specially designed test or sampling vessels with specially trained personnel. Among the vessels used in the SHAD tests were five light tugboats previously under Army command that were transferred to the Navy.

The tests using active biological agents involved selected personnel designated as Project SHAD Technical Staff (PSTS), who had security clearances and special training. PSTS manned the light tugs and the laboratory on the USS *Granville S. Hall* where the biological samples were evaluated. The light tugs had been modified to include a small laboratory and provide a positive pressure environment to limit interior exposure to test pathogens. Manned tests involving active chemical agents were carried out using the USS *George Eastman*, which had been modified in ways specifically designed to provide protection from chemical agents. Regular Navy vessels and crews were involved only in tests using simulants, not active chemical or biological agents.

As noted, a given test usually included several "trials" that were conducted over the course of days or weeks. Within a test, individual trials may have used different ships, test substances, or test conditions. Autumn Gold, for example, was conducted using four regular Navy ships and the simulant *Bacillus globigii* (BG) in nine different trials.

---

[8] In September 2011, a contract was awarded to Battelle by the Office of the Assistant Secretary of Defense for Nuclear, Chemical, and Biological Defense Programs/Chemical and Biological Defense to continue efforts of the Chemical and Biological Archive Information Management System and the U.S. Chemical and Biological Tests Repository to identify and collect Chemical and Biological Defense archival information as well as search for personnel potentially exposed to chemical agents, biological agents, or simulants while involved in tests and other ancillary events (McKim, 2013).

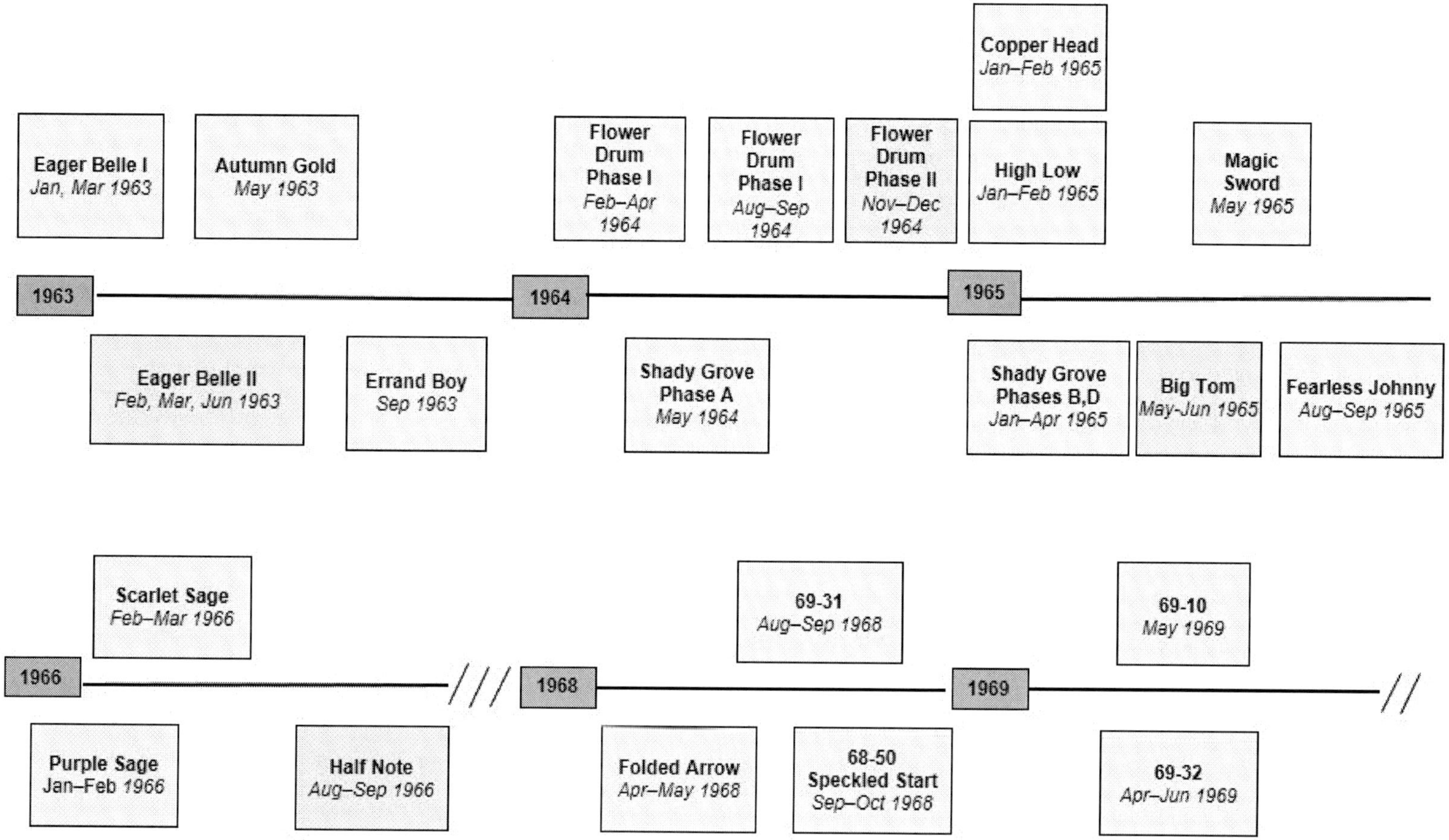


**FIGURE 2-1** Project SHAD timeline, 1963-1969.

The SHAD tests have in common that they seem to have been designed to gather operational information about the penetration of test substances into the ships, or the behavior of these substances in the specific marine environments in which they were tested. They do not have characteristics of tests carried out to evaluate the effects of the test agents on humans; such tests would presumably have included some health assessment of the study participants. In a few tests, however, samples indicating human exposure, such as gargle samples, or chemical dosimeters from clothing were collected from service members who were exposed to the test agents to evaluate personal protective equipment (Autumn Gold, DTC 69-10, Copper Head).

Three of the tests are described further here to illustrate some of the varied features of SHAD testing. A full description of each of the tests is included as an annex to this chapter.

## Autumn Gold

The Autumn Gold test (Test 63-2) was carried out in May 1963 in open sea in the Pacific Ocean approximately 60 miles west-southwest of Oahu, Hawaii. Its purpose was "to determine the degree of penetration of representative fleet ships, operating under three different material readiness conditions [ship ventilation characteristics,], by a simulant biological aerosol released from an operational weapon system" (DTC, 1964, p. iii). BG was the simulant used for this purpose. Another objective was "to estimate the magnitude and persistency [sic] of simulant biological aerosols retained after conducting air wash and hose down procedures" (DTC, 1964, p. 3). The test also provided information on the performance under the test conditions of a bacteria detector and counter and of the M17 and Mark V protective masks (DoD, 2003a).

A material readiness condition characterizes the status of ventilation settings and system access or closure on a ship. Autumn Gold was conducted in three phases of three trials each, to test the effect of material readiness conditions of Yoke, Zebra, and Zebra Circle William (DoD, 2004).[9] The participating ships were the USS *Navarro*, the USS *Tioga County*, the USS *Carpenter*, and the USS *Hoel*. In each trial, two A4B jet aircraft, each equipped with two modified Aero 14B spray tanks, disseminated BG along a single release line. For the purposes of assessing exposures for this IOM study, each release line for each trial was considered a potential exposure.

According to the final report on this test:

> Personnel on each ship were briefed on procedures for pretrial exercises and the need was stressed for attaining the three material readiness conditions during the pretrial training exercises and subsequent trials. Ship personnel conducted these exercises and inspections prior to the AUTUMN GOLD (U) trials to determine each ship's capability to fully attain these readiness conditions under its present condition…. Navy personnel from each ship were assigned to operate the various sampling equipment on the ship. These men were trained during the week prior to the first trial. (DTC, 1964, p. 7)

The test plan[10] describes procedures to test for potential for leakage of the M17 and Mark V protective masks under operational conditions using "32 test subjects (eight per ship, four at

[9] Yoke refers to routine ventilation settings in non-battle conditions. Zebra is for fire or flood control and intended to minimize water entry. Under Zebra Circle William, Circle William fittings were also closed and all ventilation fans were secured (DTC, 1965a).

[10] A test plan was a document prepared to describe planned aspects of the study in detail. It is distinct from a final report, which is intended to describe what actually took place during the test.

each of two stations per ship) … positioned at two above-deck sampling sites. Sixteen test subjects will don the M17 protective mask and 16 subjects will don the Mark V protective mask at function time and continue wearing the masks until Z+35 minutes" (DTC, 1963a, p. 74). The plan also states that those not wearing the masks would provide gargle samples before and after the test (DTC, 1963a).

Roles for a test site safety officer and medical liaison are outlined in the test plan, with the comment that "the major objective of the medical support program is to maintain the health and welfare of both military and civilian personnel while on the test site and during test operation" (DTC, 1963b, p. 80).

## Shady Grove

Most of the Shady Grove test (Test 64-4) took place in the Pacific Ocean and included a total of 25 ship-based trials that were conducted as Phases A, B, and D. Phase A was conducted in May 1964 and phases B and D during January-April 1965. (Phase C was conducted on land and is not discussed further.) Some of the Shady Grove trials used BG as a biological tracer, but other trials used the pathogenic agents *Coxiella burnetii* (referred to in the SHAD documents as OU), which causes Q fever, and *Pasteurella tularensis* (referred to as UL), which causes tularemia. Fluorescent particles (FP) of zinc cadmium sulfide were used as a tracer in all of the trials.

The stated objectives of the Shady Grove test were

> 1) To evaluate infectivity of agent UL [*Pasteurella tularensis*] aerosols over effective downwind distances, utilizing an elevated line source from an operational weapon in a marine environment. 2) To determine the viability decay of UL over effective downwind distances. 3) To characterize atmospheric diffusion in a marine environment. 4) To assess the operational capability of the weapon system. (DTC, 1965c, p. 5)

The test ships for Shady Grove were five light tugs (LTs), which carried samplers, and for some tests, animals in cages. Agents were released by a spray tank on a jet aircraft or by a disseminator mounted on one of the tugs. The USS *Granville S. Hall* served as the laboratory support ship.

Phase A was a meteorological study that included six aerial and two surface releases of BG and FP (DoD, 2004; DTC, 1965c). Phase B, in February and March 1965, included eight aerial releases of UL and BG together and one aerial release of UL only. There were also four surface releases of both UL and BG from a tug-mounted disseminator (DTC, 1965c). In the four Phase D trials, which took place between March 22 and April 3, 1965, A4C jets simultaneously disseminated BG from one tank and OU from another tank along several release lines (one aircraft per line). BG and FP were used as tracers (DTC, 1965c).

The final report indicates an awareness of safety issues and that the test was considered successful from that and other perspectives. It states that the absence of any "industrial type accidents or agent exposures" indicated an "exceptional job done in the training and execution of a test program of this magnitude" and "confirmed the feasibility of using operational combat units, with a minimum amount of personnel training and experience, to deliver biological weapons on targets from remote bases throughout the world" (DTC, 1965c).

### Flower Drum II

Although no personnel could be identified as participants in the Flower Drum II test, it is briefly described here as an example of a test that used an active chemical warfare agent. The test was carried out in the Pacific Ocean off the coast of Hawaii in November and December 1964, and included 10 trials. It was conducted to test water washdown to protect against or decontaminate after encountering an aerial spray of VX and to aid in planning a future SHAD test (DTC, 1965a). The platform for the test was the US Navy covered lighter (barge) YFN-811, which was towed by the US Navy tug ATF 105.

A spray device on the barge disseminated the test agent, which was a dyed liquid containing approximately 90 percent VX (by weight). Three conditions of water washdown were tested: (1) operating the washdown system before, during and after dissemination; (2) using the washdown immediately before and after dissemination; and (3) conducting a washdown only after dissemination was complete (DTC, 1965b).

The information available to the committee does not indicate that any people were aboard the barge during the test. Because no deck logs were found for either vessel, no veterans who may have participated in the test could be identified and included in the analysis for either the SHAD I study or the current study.

## PREVIOUS STUDIES OF SHAD VETERANS

Two previous studies have investigated the health outcomes and health status of SHAD veterans. One study (Kang and Bullman, 2009) was conducted by VA personnel. The other was the previous study conducted at the IOM (2007). Both studies are briefly reviewed here.

### VA Study of SHAD Veterans

Kang and Bullman (2009) carried out a study of mortality in the Navy SHAD veteran population. In their study, 4,927 SHAD study participants and a comparison veteran population were followed to date of death or December 31, 2004, whichever was earlier. The comparison population of veterans who did not participate in SHAD tests was a stratified random sample of 10,927 men drawn from a group of 164,277 male Vietnam-era veterans who served in the Navy between 1962 and 1973 (the time frame for the SHAD tests). The control subjects were selected using birth-year strata to provide a roughly 2-to-1 match with the SHAD veterans. Within the population of SHAD veterans, the researchers also compared the veterans who were exposed to active biological or chemical agents with those who were only exposed to simulants or tracers. The study found a statistically significant increased risk of overall mortality among SHAD veterans (an all-cause adjusted rate ratio [ARR] of 1.10, 95% confidence interval [CI] 1.01-1.97), with the excess mortality due primarily to heart disease (heart disease ARR 1.39, 95% CI 1.18-1.64). The increased risk was observed only in those SHAD veterans who were exposed to simulants, not in those potentially exposed to active chemical or biological agents. No other excess in cause-specific mortality was observed among SHAD veterans.

### The IOM's Previous Study of SHAD Veterans

In 2002, the IOM was asked to conduct a study to assess whether SHAD veterans might be experiencing adverse health conditions that could be associated with their participation in

Project SHAD. The IOM study chose a different strategy for selection of a comparison group for the study. Completed in 2007, the IOM's SHAD I study compared the morbidity and mortality experience of SHAD veterans with that of a population of crew members of ships selected to match the ships that had participated in each SHAD test.[11] This approach to the selection of a comparison population was used to attempt to ensure that members of the study population had service at sea (or in a similar Marine unit) at a similar time and in a similar geographic area, making inclusion in the SHAD tests a principal point of difference.

The IOM researchers assembled a roster of 5,867 Project SHAD veterans (test participants) and a comparison population of 6,757 Navy and Marine Corps personnel (controls) (IOM, 2007). Mortality data (including cause of death after 1979) were obtained from VA and the files of the National Death Index. Of the nearly 12,500 Navy and Marine Corps study subjects, approximately 9,600 were assumed to be alive as of December 31, 2004 (i.e., there was no evidence of death from available records sources).

The surviving participants and controls who could be located were asked to complete a health survey by mail or telephone. The survey included general demographic information and questions about smoking, weight, and alcohol use in order to have information about important influences on health status. It included portions of validated tests of physical symptoms and well-being in the form of the physical and mental health status components of the Short Form 36 Health Survey (SF-36). It also included a standard list of medical conditions and symptoms for self-report, and a scale for assessing neurological problems and cognitive difficulties. Veterans of SHAD testing were asked additional questions about any symptoms experienced during the tests, use of protective gear during the tests, and experience with decontamination. Also included were several questions from a survey that SHAD veterans had designed and circulated as health concerns were first coming to light. Mail questionnaire or telephone interview responses were received from 61 percent of Project SHAD participants and 47 percent of controls.

The study included analyses of mortality and morbidity. Both standardized mortality ratios (SMRs) and proportional hazards modeling were used to analyze mortality. The covariates included in the analyses were participant status, SHAD participant exposure group, age, race, branch of service, pay grade, rank, length of service, vital status, date of death, and cause of death. The primary health outcome for the morbidity analysis was the score on the SF-36 assessment of general health. Also used were scores on two subscales of the SF-36: for the physical component summary (PCS) and mental component summary (MCS). Other outcome variables derived from the health survey included a history of medical conditions, present symptoms, and hospitalizations after completion of military service.

Many of the analyses grouped Project SHAD participants into four broad exposure categories to evaluate whether health outcomes differed by specific patterns of exposure. Group A, with roughly 3,400 participants, was exposed only to BG or methylacetoacetate (MAA). In group B were the roughly 900 participants exposed to trioctyl phosphate (TOF) in Test 69-10. Group C included the approximately 750 participants who were potentially exposed to active chemical or biological agents, with or without possible additional exposure to simulants. Group D—870 participants—included the men who did not meet the criteria for the other three categories. Their exposures may have included BG or MAA in combination with other simulants or tracers or decontaminants; none of the men in Group D were exposed to active agents or TOF.

The study found no difference in all-cause mortality between Project SHAD participants and controls, although participants had a statistically significantly higher risk of death due to

[11] The selection of the ships for the comparison population is described in detail in Chapter 3.

heart disease (hazard ratio [HR] = 1.20, 95% CI, 1.03-1.39). The lack of data on cardiovascular risk factors or any explanation as to the biological plausibility of the association made the heart disease results difficult to interpret. Participants were also found to have reported statistically significantly worse health than controls as measured by the PCS and the MCS scores on the SF-36 portion of the questionnaire, but no consistent, specific, clinically significant patterns of ill health were found. The group with potential exposure to active chemical or biological agents had the most positive SF-36 health score among the four exposure groups. There were small but statistically significant increases in self-reported memory and attention problems in three of the exposure groups and in somatization scores for all participants. The full group of Project SHAD participants reported higher levels of neurodegenerative medical conditions compared with the control group, but most of these conditions were of an unspecified nature. Participants also reported nearly uniformly higher rates of various symptoms. However, higher rates of a symptom without an apparent medical basis (earlobe pain) suggested the possibility of reporting bias. The SHAD participants and controls had no significant differences in self-reported hospitalizations. Although the participants in one of the exposure groups reported a higher rate of birth defects than controls, this statistically significant difference was attributed to an unusually low rate of birth defects among the control group rather than to a higher rate among participants.[12]

While the SHAD I study found no clear evidence of specific health effects associated with participation in Project SHAD, the authors noted that the results do not constitute clear evidence of a lack of health effects. Some of the exposure groups were moderate in size, and the lack of specific a priori hypotheses of health effects was a limitation. If there were, for example, very specific but relatively infrequent effects on a particular organ system, the study's broad groupings of health outcomes might have obscured such a specific effect.

### Supplemental SHAD I Analyses

In February 2008 Congressmen Mike Thompson and Dennis Rehberg, who had received a briefing on the SHAD I study, directed five follow-up questions to the IOM. These questions requested additional information or clarification on the personnel who were included or excluded in the analysis, the availability of information on health outcomes for some SHAD participants, the potential impact of duty assignments on exposures of SHAD participants, and characterizations of the SHAD tests. In August 2008, IOM staff responded to these questions with comments and supplemental analyses (IOM, 2008).

The analysis included crews of the light tugs (104 men) for only one test (Shady Grove) because rosters for tug crews during other tests could not be located by DoD or through independent efforts by the IOM staff. No other means was found to identify crewmembers from these vessels. Conversely, the congressional questions also reflected concern that the crews of the USS *Granville S. Hall* and the USS *George Eastman* had less exposure than other SHAD participants and that their inclusion in the analysis could have obscured associations with adverse health outcomes. Supplemental analyses that separated the crews of these two ships found that all-cause mortality and self-reported physical health of the other SHAD participants was "essentially the same as the published results of analyses that included these personnel" (IOM,

[12] The self-reported rate of birth defects among group D participants was similar to the rate in the other participant groups; whereas, the self-reported rate among the controls for group D was markedly lower (IOM, 2007).

2008). There were, however, indications of higher mortality and poorer health status among the crew of the USS *George Eastman* when they were analyzed separately (IOM, 2008).

The supplemental report also reviewed the SHAD I efforts to identify all deaths among SHAD veterans and the cause of death for all deaths from 1979 through 2004. Determining causes of the 357 deaths that occurred before 1979 was not considered feasible during the SHAD I study, but obtaining as much of this information as possible was a specific priority for the SHAD II study. The lack of explicit information on crew members' tasks or locations during tests and the IOM's efforts to solicit information about the tests from SHAD veterans were both reiterated in the supplemental report. As has been noted, these concerns were a motivation in the SHAD II study to specifically develop new ways to incorporate information about likely variations in exposure in the analysis.

## CONCERNS EXPRESSED BY SHAD VETERANS

An express element of the legislation that requested the IOM's SHAD II study was that a public workshop be organized to ensure veteran input to inform the conduct of the study. The IOM Committee on Shipboard Hazard and Defense II held two public meetings at which SHAD veterans had an opportunity to speak to the committee. At the first meeting, statements from eight veterans helped introduce committee members to Project SHAD. At a second meeting, held in Sacramento, California, the committee heard from three panels that each included four to six veterans who spoke about their experiences during various SHAD tests, their health concerns, and their perspectives regarding key information sources or approaches to the study. The committee also received written statements submitted by other veterans who did not attend the meetings, and several veterans spoke with members of the committee staff over the course of the study.

The comments offered by SHAD veterans provided helpful insights and observations. It was clear that veterans' experiences in the tests varied widely and that generalizations across the tests or the participating ships are difficult because the nature of the tests, test agents, and ship settings varied. However, some themes that emerged from the veterans' remarks are described here.

### Information Limitations

At the time of Project SHAD, the tests were classified as Top Secret or Secret and information about them was highly compartmentalized. Even the men who served as part of the Project SHAD Technical Staff on the light tugs, the USS *Granville S. Hall*, or the USS *George Eastman* were not given information about the purpose, operational details, or results of a test beyond what they needed to carry out their specific tasks. They were not permitted to keep any relevant records after completion of their tasks or tests. On other ships, some sailors recalled being briefed by their commanders about the ship's participation in a chemical or biological weapons exercise, while others recalled no warning before their ship was sprayed with a substance unknown to them. In other cases, some SHAD veterans were keenly aware that they were participants in simulant testing because they wore dosimeters to evaluate their exposure to the test agent or thermometers to monitor their physical status while wearing protective gear. Several of the veterans remembered strong admonitions not to share information about the tests, with threats of severe punishment for violators.

Some of the veterans who spoke to the committee also noted gaps or missing items in their medical records. For example, certain of the PSTS veterans recalled being given multiple vaccinations (e.g., against tularemia, Q fever, and Venezuelan equine encephalitis) prior to their involvement in tests of biological agents. However, the veterans reported that these vaccinations were not recorded in their regular medical records when those records were retrieved years later (Testimony to IOM Committee on Shipboard Hazard and Defense II, February 2012). Similarly, a veteran who remembered several visits to sick bay during the time of the test he was involved in found no record of these medical visits when he requested and received his medical records from the Navy (Personal communication, G. Arnold, SHAD veteran, USS *Navarro*, Sacramento, California, February 23, 2012). Limited access to detailed information about the SHAD tests continues to be a concern to veterans. As noted in Chapter 1, many of the operational details of the tests remain classified; only report pages deemed "medically relevant" were declassified and made public (Morris, 2004). Veterans at the committee's workshop questioned the need for continued secrecy regarding details of the tests and their results because the types of ships that were used are no longer in the Navy's fleet.

Because of the limitations of the information that has been declassified, veterans must rely on their recollections from the 1960s to fill in details beyond the information available in the DoD Fact Sheets and the redacted technical documents. As several veterans acknowledged, it is difficult to be definitive about events from that period.

Because the available information is limited, at least some veterans expressed concerns about the committee's ability to refine assessments of exposure beyond the steps taken in the IOM SHAD I study. This issue is discussed further in Chapter 3, Study Approach and Design.

### Involuntary Participation

Another concern is the involuntary nature of their participation in the tests. Although participation as a member of the PSTS was nominally voluntary, it took place within the command structure of military service. The regular crew members of the ships involved in the testing and the Marines in participating units reported no options regarding participation, including in particular those who were identified to provide gargle samples or run sampling stations.

### Uninformed VA Staff

Veterans expressed to the committee and the IOM staff their ongoing frustration with the lack of knowledge about the SHAD tests in the VA health care system. Public Law 110-387, the Veterans' Mental Health and Other Care Improvement Act of 2008, provided for veterans who participated in Project 112 (which included the SHAD tests) to be enrolled in Priority Group 6 for health care at the Veterans Health Administration (VHA).[13] As a result, VA issued a directive (VHA, 2009, 2015) that these veterans "are eligible to receive needed VA hospital care, medical services, and may be provided nursing home care for any illness notwithstanding insufficient medical evidence to conclude that such illness is attributable to such testing. No copayments apply to the receipt of this care" (VHA, 2015, p. 1). The VHA 2009 policy called for these

[13] VA established Priority Groups as a means to make sure that some groups of veterans are able to be enrolled before others. Priority Groups range from 1 to 8, with 1 the highest priority for enrollment. Eligibility for Priority grouping takes into account factors such as the extent of service-connected disability, employment, receipt of various medals, and income (VA, 2015).

veterans to be offered "a thorough clinical evaluation by a knowledgeable VA primary care provider; enhanced priority for enrollment in the VA Health Care System; and pertinent information about Project 112 SHAD exposures and possible related adverse health effects" (VHA, 2009, p. 2). Nevertheless, SHAD veterans reported continuing to encounter VA health care providers who had not heard of SHAD and therefore do not have an appropriate context for evaluating health issues brought to them by the veterans.

SHAD veterans seeking disability benefits from VA also expressed frustration about the need to document their participation in Project SHAD even though security procedures did not permit them to keep records or other documentation when a test was completed. The SHAD veterans contrast their circumstances with those of veterans who served in Vietnam who are presumed to have been exposed to Agent Orange when they are seeking to qualify for a service-connected disability for one of the conditions that has been defined as associated with Agent Orange exposure. The SHAD veterans had unwitting or at least often involuntary participation in tests of chemical or biological agents or simulants and see justification for establishing a presumption that their participation in these tests qualifies them for service-connected disabilities. There is currently no finding of specific conditions associated with SHAD exposures, however, and that is an impetus for the research questions for this study.

Members of the PSTS had a unique experience within the SHAD tests, and they have a special set of concerns. These men participated in tests that used not only simulants and related test substances but also active biological agents. In addition, many of these men had unusual working conditions as a result of serving as crewmen on the five light tug boats that had been refitted to be used as sampling stations. PSTS members noted to the committee that these tugs were designed for service in a harbor and not in the open ocean where SHAD tests were conducted.

## CONCLUDING REMARKS

Project SHAD included a diverse set of tests conducted during a 7-year period in which more than 21 Navy vessels, several Marine ground units, and at least eight Marine or Navy air units participated in some manner. An understanding of the nature and diversity of the tests, gained from both veterans and DoD documents, was important in helping the committee frame its approach to the analysis of the available data on test exposures and health outcomes. Chapter 3 reviews several issues that were important in shaping the analysis.

## REFERENCES

Beard, V. L. 1996. *Letter to Mel Hancock, U.S. House of Representatives.* October 28, Washington, DC: Special Actions Branch, Department of the Army.

DoD (Department of Defense). 2003a. *Deseret Test Center, Project SHAD: Autumn Gold (Update).* Factsheet, Version 12-2-2003. Washington, DC: The Office of the Assistant Secretary of Defense (Health Affairs), Deployment Health Support Directorate. http://mcm.fhpr.osd.mil/Libraries/CBexposuresDocs/autumn_gold_revised.sflb.ashx (accessed May 13, 2014).

DoD. 2003b. *Deseret Test Center, Project SHAD: DTC Test 70-C.* Factsheet, Version 6-30-2003. Washington, DC: The Office of the Assistant Secretary of Defense (Health Affairs), Deployment Health Support Directorate. http://mcm.fhpr.osd.mil/Libraries/CBexposuresDocs/dtc_test_70_C.sflb.ashx (accessed January 13, 2015).

DoD. 2003c. *2003 Report to Congress: Disclosure of information on Project 112 to the Department of Veterans Affairs as directed by PL 107-314.* Washington, DC: Office of the Assistant Secretary of Defense (Health Affairs).

DoD. 2004 (unpublished). *SHAD test information.* Provided to the Institute of Medicine in response to an information request submitted by Susanne Stoiber, Executive Officer, Institute of Medicine, to William Winkenwerder, Assistant Secretary of Defense for Health Affairs, Department of Defense. Washington, DC.

DoD. 2011. *Release from "secrecy oaths" under chemical and biological weapons human subject research programs.* Memorandum from William J. Lynn III, Deputy Secretary of Defense, January 11. http://mcm.fhpr.osd.mil/Libraries/CBexposuresDocs/OSD_14995-10.sflb.ashx (accessed January 14, 2014).

DoD. 2014. *Project 112/SHAD—Shipboard Hazard and Defense.* http://mcm.fhpr.osd.mil/cb_exposures/project112_shad/shad.aspx (accessed January 3, 2014).

DoD. 2015. *Project 112/SHAD fact sheets.* http://www.health.mil/Military-Health-Topics/Health-Readiness/Environmental-Exposures/Project-112-SHAD/Fact-Sheets (accessed October 15, 2015).

DTC (Deseret Test Center). 1963a. *Autumn Gold (U). Revision 1, Test Plan 63-2, April 1963, Appendix H, Defensive Tests, Part I.* Redacted excerpts. Fort Douglas, UT: Deseret Test Center.

DTC 1963b. *Autumn Gold (U), Revision 1, Test Plan 63-2, April 1963, Appendix K.* Redacted excerpts. Fort Douglas, UT: Deseret Test Center.

DTC. 1964. *Autumn Gold (U). Test 63-2, Final Report, May 1964.* Redacted excerpts. Fort Douglas, UT: Deseret Test Center.

DTC. 1965a. *Test 64-2—Flower Drum (U), Phase I.* Final report—Revised. December. Redacted excerpts from pp. cover, iii, iv, 3-5, 7-9, 11, 13, 20, 22, 28, 57, 63. Rpt. No. DTC 642110R. Fort Douglas, UT: Deseret Test Center.

DTC. 1965b. *Test 64-2, Flower Drum (U), Phase II, Final Report, October 1965.* Report Number DTC 642105R. Redacted excerpts. Fort Douglas, UT: Deseret Test Center.

DTC. 1965c. *Test 64-4 Shady Grove (U), Final Report, December 1965.* Redacted excerpts. Headquarters, Fort Douglas, UT: Deseret Test Center.

EPA (Environmental Protection Agency). 2014. *Clean Air Act requirements and history.* http://www.epa.gov/air/caa/requirements.html (accessed January 14, 2014).

GAO (General Accounting Office). 2004. *Chemical and biological defense: DoD needs to continue to collect and provide information on tests and potentially exposed personnel.* GAO-04-410. Washington, DC: General Accounting Office.

GAO (Government Accountability Office). 2008. *Chemical and biological defense: DoD and VA need to improve efforts to identify and notify individuals potentially exposed during chemical and biological tests.* GAO-08-366. Washington, DC: Government Accountability Office.

Gober, H. W. 2000. *Letter to William S. Cohen, Secretary, Department of Defense.* August 3, Washington, DC: Department of Veterans Affairs.

IOM (Institute of Medicine). 2007. *Long-term health effects of participation in Project SHAD (Shipboard Hazard and Defense).* Washington, DC: The National Academies Press.

IOM. 2008. *Response to 15 February 2008 letter from Congressmen Mike Thompson and Dennis Rehberg.* http://iom.nationalacademies.org/~/media/Files/Report%20Files/2007/Long-Term-Health-Effects-of-Participation-in-Project-SHAD-Shipboard-Hazard-and-Defense/SHAD%20Response%20Letter.pdf (accessed October 7, 2015).

Kang, H. K., and T. Bullman. 2009. Mortality follow-up of veterans who participated in military chemical and biological warfare agent testing between 1962 and 1972. *Journal of Toxicology and Environmental Health, Part A* 72:1550-1552.

McKim, W. D. 2013. *Interim technical report on CBAIMS and U.S. Chemical and Biological Tests Repository from September 2011-May 2013.* Washington, DC: Batelle.

Morris, D. D. 2004. *The Department of Defense identification of participants and exposures in Projects 112 and Shipboard Hazard and Defense.* M.P.H. Thesis, Morris, Dee Dodson: George Washington University.

Murphy, J. 2003. *Secrecy over Cold War WMD tests.* CBS News, July 1. http://www.cbsnews.com/news/secrecy-over-cold-war-wmd-tests (accessed January 13, 2015).

Nixon, R. 1969. *Remarks announcing decisions on chemical and biological defense policies and programs.* November 25. Online by G. Peters and J. T. Woolley, The American Presidency Project. http://www.presidency.ucsb.edu/ws/?pid=2344 (accessed January 14, 2014).

VA (Department of Veterans Affairs). 2015. *Health benefits: Priority groups.* http://www.va.gov/HEALTHBENEFITS/resources/priority_groups.asp (accessed January 21, 2015).

VHA (Veterans Health Administration). 2009. *Provision of health care services to veterans involved in Project 112-Shipboard Hazard and Defense (SHAD) Testing.* VHA Directive 2009-047, September 30. Washington, DC: Veterans Health Administration, Department of Veterans Affairs.

VHA. 2015. *Provision of health care services to veterans involved in Project 112-Shipboard and Land-based Hazard and Defense Testing (Project 112/SHAD).* VHA Directive 1127, March 24. Washington, DC: Veterans Health Administration, Department of Veterans Affairs.

# Annex

# Brief Descriptions of SHAD Tests

The Department of Defense (DoD) has identified 21 Project SHAD tests that were conducted between 1963 and 1973. A total of 39 tests had been planned for Project SHAD, but 18 tests were cancelled. The summaries that follow describe essential features of each of the tests that were conducted. This information is drawn from redacted technical and final reports on the tests that have been made public, from the DoD Fact Sheets for each test that were based on those materials,[1] and from spreadsheets with additional detail on the trials within each test that were provided to the Institute of Medicine by DoD (DoD, 2004). Where the information is available, each summary provides the name, dates, location, number of trials, substances used, and ships involved. Procedures, use of decontaminants, or use of protective gear are noted when that information was reported in the available documents. The tests are presented in the order in which they took place and the source documents are listed with each test summary.

*These descriptions closely follow or quote the original technical reports or other sources where indicated.*

**Eager Belle I (Test 63-1)**

*January, March 1963*

The Eager Belle I test consisted of 17 exposure trials and was carried out in the Pacific Ocean west of Oahu, Hawaii. The test was intended "to evaluate the effectiveness of selected protective devices in preventing penetration of a naval ship by a biological aerosol," and "to compare the efficiency of the M-17 and the Mark V protective masks against a biological aerosol" (DTC, 1965, p. iii).

The test used *Bacillus globigii* (BG),[2] and the test ship was the USS *George Eastman*. For each of 17 trials (9 in January, 8 in March), BG was disseminated from the stern of a tugboat over a 10-minute period. Fog oil was also discharged to provide a visible tracer of the release. The *George Eastman* steamed 500 yards behind the tugboat, striving to remain within the aerosol

[1] The DoD Fact Sheets for Project SHAD tests (and Project 112 tests) are available at http://www.health.mil/Military-Health-Topics/Health-Readiness/Environmental-Exposures/Project-112-SHAD/Fact-Sheets (accessed September 23, 2015).

[2] The majority of the SHAD tests involved use of an aerosol containing the organism referred to then—and in this report—as *Bacillus globigii* (BG). This organism has also been known as *Bacillus subtilis var. niger* and is currently typically referred to as *Bacillus atrophaeus*.

cloud. Trials were carried out under four different ventilation conditions. Samplers were positioned on the exterior and interior of the ship to evaluate penetration of the aerosol under the different ventilation conditions.

*Source:*

DTC (Deseret Test Center). 1965. *Eager Belle (U), Phase I (Revised).* DTC Final Report, Test 63-1. 30 June. Redacted excerpts from cover, pp. iii, iv, 5, 6, 37-39, 70. DMMC Control #2001235-0000009, DMMC Control #2000300-0000012. Fort Douglas, UT: Deseret Test Center.

**Eager Belle II**

*February, March, June 1963*

The Eager Belle Phase II test consisted of 14 exposure trials and was conducted in the Pacific Ocean, roughly 175 miles west of Oahu, Hawaii. BG was used to study the downwind travel of biological aerosols. Testers sought "to relate biological aerosol cloud travel to predicted cloud travel based on present prediction models for prevailing conditions," "to obtain additional information on weapon system performance … over the open sea under the meteorological conditions encountered," and "to obtain information to assist in the design and execution of future trials" (DTC, n.d., p. 2). An additional objective was to evaluate, in environmental conditions, the performance of a particle-size analyzer that was under development.

For Eager Belle Phase II trials, BG was released as a line source generated by Aero 14B spray tanks mounted on A4 series jet attack aircraft. For the first 11 trials, the USS *George Eastman* was the test ship and carried the sampling devices. For the last three trials, the samplers were aboard the USS *Navarro*, USS *Tioga County*, and USS *Carpenter*, all of which participated in the three trials. Trials included downwind testing at short and longer distances from the line source. The operating conditions of the ships were not recorded in the final report but were inferred to be Zebra by those at DoD who reviewed the reports in 2004 (DoD, 2004).

*Sources:*

DoD (Department of Defense). 2004 (unpublished). *SHAD test information.* Provided to the Institute of Medicine in response to an information request submitted by Susanne Stoiber, Executive Officer, Institute of Medicine, to William Winkenwerder, Assistant Secretary of Defense for Health Affairs, Department of Defense. Washington, DC.

DTC. n.d. *Eager Belle, Phase 2.* DCT Test 63-1, Technical Report. Redacted excerpts from pages iii, iv, 2-5. Distributed by Defense Technical Information Center, Alexandria, VA.

**Autumn Gold (Test 63-2)**

*May 1963*

The Autumn Gold test was carried out in open sea in the Pacific Ocean approximately 60 miles west-southwest of Oahu, Hawaii, and it used BG as a test substance. Its purpose was "to determine the degree of penetration of representative fleet ships, operating under three different material readiness conditions, by a simulant biological aerosol released from an operational weapon system" (DTC, 1964, p. iii). Another objective was "to estimate the magnitude and persistency of simulant biological aerosols retained after conducting air wash and hose down procedures" (DTC, 1964, p. 3). The test also provided information on the performance of equipment, including the M17 and Mark V protective masks (DTC, 1964, p. 3).

The test included nine trials and was conducted in three phases of three trials each, testing the Yoke, Zebra, and Zebra Circle William material conditions (DoD, 2004). The participating ships were the USS *Navarro*, USS *Tioga County*, USS *Carpenter*, and USS *Hoel*. The USS *Hoel* did not participate in the last two trials. In each trial, two A4B jet aircraft, each equipped with two modified Aero 14B spray tanks, disseminated BG along a release line.

According to the final report, "Personnel on each ship were briefed on procedures for pretrial exercises and the need was stressed for attaining the three material readiness conditions during the pretrial training exercises and subsequent trials. Ship personnel conducted these exercises and inspections prior to the AUTUMN GOLD (U) trials to determine each ship's capability to fully attain these readiness conditions under its present condition.... Navy personnel from each ship were assigned to operate the various sampling equipment on the ship. These men were trained during the week prior to the first trial" (DTC, 1964, p. 7).

The following procedures to test for potential for leakage of the M17 and Mark V protective masks under operational conditions were described in the test plan: "In each trial of AUTUMN GOLD, 32 test subjects (eight per ship, four at each of two stations per ship) will be positioned at two above deck sampling sites. Sixteen test subjects will don the M17 protective mask and 16 subjects will don the Mark V protective mask at function time and continue wearing the masks until Z+35 minutes [35 minutes after release]" (DTC, 1963, p. 74).

The test plan also states that "all test subjects not wearing the oronasal mask and all test subject controls will provide a gargle sample prior to function time and again immediately after Z+35 minutes. All gargle samples and the oronasal masks will be assayed on the laboratory ship YAG 40. Leakage of the protective masks will be determined by analysis of the data" (DTC, 1963, p. 74).

Roles for a test site safety officer and medical liaison are outlined in the test plan, with the comment that "the major objective of the medical support program is to maintain the health and welfare of both military and civilian personnel while on the test site and during test operation" (DTC, 1963, p. 80).

*Sources:*

DTC. 1963. *Autumn Gold (U).* Test Plan 63-2, Revision 1, April. Redacted excerpts from cover, pp. 2, 7, 9, 11, 12, 14-16, 21, 23, 31, 74, 77, 79-81, 86-91, 93-95. AD 352693. Fort Douglas, UT: Deseret Test Center.

DTC. 1964. *Autumn Gold (U).* DTC Final Report, Test 63-2. May. Redacted excerpts from cover, pp. i, iii, v-x, unnumbered drawing, 1-3, 5-7, A1-A4, D1-D2, E1-E2, F1-F4. AD 350542-064. Fort Douglas, UT: Deseret Test Center.

**Errand Boy (Test 64-1)**

*September 1963*

Errand Boy was carried out aboard the USS *George Eastman* while it was moored at Buoy X-9 in East Loch, Pearl Harbor, Hawaii. Errand Boy was originally designed as an extension of the Eager Belle and Autumn Gold tests to obtain similar data about the relative efficiency of shipboard collective protection and ventilation systems, using the pathogenic test agents *Pasteurella tularensis* (*P. tularensis*, now designated *Francisella tularensis*) and Venezuelan equine encephalomyelitis virus instead of BG (DoD, 2003).

The original objectives of Errand Boy were to determine the degree to which "biological agent aerosols penetrate a ship's interior and the extent of any associated surface contamination hazard under various combinations of shipboard collective protection and ventilation systems; and to evaluate the effectiveness of various decontamination procedures for decontaminating exterior surfaces" (DoD, 2003). The penetration phase of the test was not conducted; as a result, the biological agents *P. tularensis* and Venezuelan equine encephalomyelitis virus were not disseminated.

Planning for the use of pathogenic biological agents for Errand Boy also included planning for decontamination. An engineering survey of the USS *George Eastman* was conducted by representatives of the Deseret Test Center (DTC), Chemical Research and Development Laboratories (CRDL), Naval Biological Laboratories (NBL), Project SHAD Technical Staff, and the USS *George Eastman*. Following the survey, modifications were made to the ship's air circulation and ventilation system at Pearl Harbor Naval Shipyard. Systems qualification tests were carried out both in port and at sea in July and August 1963 (DTC, 1965).

Between September 6 and 17, eight decontamination trials were carried out "to attempt a demonstration of the effectiveness of betapropiolactone (BPL) as a disinfectant for the interior spaces of the ship" (DTC, 1965, p. 2). For each of the trials, patches impregnated with known numbers of BG microorganisms were placed in the zone of the ship being tested. BPL was used for the decontamination, with a standard dissemination time of 80 minutes in each zone (DoD, 2003). Personnel who were to enter areas with high concentrations of BPL vapor wore impermeable (rubber) clothing, and the test zones were closed to all other personnel (DoD, 2003; DTC, 1965, p. 17). The test location was selected to avoid downwind hazard to the shore in Hawaii (DTC, 1965).

After the BPL testing was completed, the medical and safety officer had to certify that air in the zone being decontaminated was free of BPL and safe to reoccupy for normal operations. (DTC, 1965).

*Sources:*

DoD. 2003. *Fact sheet: Errand Boy,* version 06-30-2003. http://www.health.mil/Reference-Center/Fact-Sheets/2003/06/30/Errand-Boy (accessed September 23, 2015).

DTC. 1965. *Observations on ship decontamination (U).* Technical Memorandum. November. Redacted excerpts from cover, abstract, pp. 2, 5, 6, 8, 16, 17, 32, 33. DMMC Control #2003154-0000031. Fort Douglas, UT: Deseret Test Center.

### Flower Drum I (Test 64-2)

*February-April, August-September 1964*

The Flower Drum test was "designed to find a simulant for agent GB [sarin nerve agent], to assess shipboard vulnerability to an enveloping vapor of toxic agent, and to establish comparative penetration properties for [sarin nerve agent] simulant and agent" (DTC, 1965, p. iii). It included 31 trials and took place in the Pacific Ocean off the coast of Hawaii. The test ship was the USS *George Eastman*, which was described as a "specially designed and equipped test ship" (DTC, 1965, p. iii). The USS *Granville S. Hall* participated as an escort ship and laboratory resource.

Five initial trials were carried out between February and April 1964 and used sulfur dioxide ($SO_2$) as a simulant (DoD, 2004; DTC, 1965, p. iv). After investigation of other simulant candidates, methyl acetoacetate (MAA) was selected and used in comprehensive, comparative trials during August and September 1964. Twenty-six trials used either the simulant MAA, sarin, or a combination of MAA and sarin, and of these, nine trials used sarin nerve agent (DoD, 2004; DTC, 1965, pp. 22, 57).

The Flower Drum test involved evaluation of four test conditions and specific installed protective systems. Additional objectives for the Flower Drum test were to report information applicable to the Navy's Chemical Training Program, and to obtain information on the performance of the E41 V-G agent alarm system, the hydrogen flame emission detector (HYFED) candidate point sampling alarms, and the passive long path infrared (LOPAIR) advance warning alarm (each modified for shipboard use) when exposed to a cloud of sarin nerve agent (DTC, 1965).

The final report on the test outlines the procedures for the trials (DTC, 1965). The USS *George Eastman* "steamed into the wind maintaining a relative wind speed of 10 to 30 knots. The [USS *Granville S. Hall*] maintained a parallel course forward and starboard of the [USS *George Eastman*]" (DTC, 1965, p. 11). Sarin nerve agent or a simulant ($SO_2$ or MAA) was released only when the appropriate material condition was set and all personnel except the disseminator crew were within the safety citadel (a specially designated area of the test ship). The sarin or a stimulant was disseminated for 10 minutes at a rate that maintained an average concentration of approximately 50 mg/m$^3$ at the forward deckhouse bulkhead. Dissemination was via a gas turbine on the bow or direct injection into the ventilation system intake.

During dissemination of sarin nerve agent, "the disseminator crew wore M5 protective ensembles and all other personnel (who were in the safety citadel) wore MK5, M7A1, or M17 protective masks. After dissemination, all personnel whose duties required them to leave the safety citadel wore protective masks until the ship was cleared of [sarin]. During the dissemination period of the simulant trials, all personnel wore protective masks" (DTC, 1965, p. 11).

The report on the test also states, "During test periods, the only entrance to or exit from the safety citadel was through a decontamination tunnel, which consisted of a passageway that functioned as an air-sweep tunnel for the decontamination facility and also as one of two primary ventilation exhausts for the safety citadel. The passageway was divided into four sections by perforated doors; the doors restricted the rate of airflow and maintained the interior/exterior pressure differential. The decontamination tunnel was outfitted with a gas chamber to be used [to check protective masks], shower facilities (not used during the test of vapor agents), and protective equipment and clothing removal facilities. All personnel worked in teams (or two or more persons), and all teams were checked in and out of the safety citadel" (DTC, 1965, p. 13).

Following the completion of sampling, the ship was fully aerated. For the sarin nerve agent trials, "aeration of the ship was continued until the enzyme ticket test of the M15A1 detector kit indicated there was no [sarin nerve agent] in the exhaust air" (DTC, 1965, p. 20). At that point, "properly protected personnel confirmed the absence of [sarin] within each area" by using the enzyme ticket test of the M15A1 detector kit (DTC, 1965, p. 20).

Additional information regarding training and equipment from the Flower Drum Phase I Final Report:

> a. <u>Ship's Crew Training Program</u>: A detailed training program was administered to the ships' companies (which were specially selected) … prior to the beginning of trials. The training program was [SHAD] oriented but gave fundamental training in basic [chemical warfare/weapons] CW principles. The results of the training were satisfactory; the crews

were adequately prepared, and refresher and supplementary information and materials were not required. …

b. Protective Gear:

(1) With regard to the M5 protective ensemble worn by the disseminator crew, the following was reported:

(a) … Because of the fragile character of certain M5 ensemble components, extreme care should be used in its handling and storage.

(b) Life support systems utilizing cryogenic liquid oxygen might prove invaluable in the tactical applications of CW weapons in the field. Elimination of "umbilical" type attachments would provide greater freedom of movement.

(2) Protective masks were worn by all personnel during all [sarin] trials; personnel in the Safety Citadel wore masks during dissemination and until the disseminator was cleared of agent. During the series of trials, MK5, M7A1, and M17 protective masks were used and found to be satisfactory; no recommendation is made. (DTC, 1965, p. 63)

*Sources:*

DoD. 2004 (unpublished). *SHAD test information.* Provided to the Institute of Medicine in response to an information request submitted by Susanne Stoiber, Executive Officer, Institute of Medicine, to William Winkenwerder, Assistant Secretary of Defense for Health Affairs, Department of Defense. Washington, DC.

DTC. 1965. *Test 64-2—Flower Drum (U), Phase I.* Final report—Revised. December. Redacted excerpts from cover, pp. iii, iv, 3-5, 7-9, 11, 13, 20, 22, 28, 57, 63. Rpt. No. DTC 642110R. Fort Douglas, UT: Deseret Test Center.

**Shady Grove (Test 64-4)**

*Phase A: May 1964*

*Phases B, D: January-April 1965*

The Shady Grove test took place in the Pacific Ocean and included a total of 25 ship-based trials that were conducted as Phases A, B, and D. (Phase C was conducted on land and is not discussed further here.) In addition to use of BG as a simulant for a biological warfare agent, the test included trials with the pathogenic agents *Coxiella burnetii* (OU), which causes Q fever, and *Pasteurella tularensis* (UL), which causes tularemia. Fluorescent particles of zinc cadmium sulfide (FP) were used as a tracer.

The stated objectives of the Shady Grove test were "1) To evaluate infectivity of *Pasteurella tularensis* (UL) aerosols over effective downwind distances, utilizing an elevated line source from an operational weapon in a marine environment. 2) To determine the viability decay of UL over effective downwind distances. 3) To characterize atmospheric diffusion in a marine environment. 4) To assess the operational capability of the weapon system" (DTC, 1965, p. 5).

The test ships for Shady Grove were five Army light tugs (LTs) (hull numbers 2080, 2081, 2085, 2086, and 2087), which carried samplers. For 19 of the trials, the test agents were released by an Aero 14B spray tank mounted on an A4C jet aircraft system, and in six trials the agents were released on the surface by a multi-nozzle E-2 disseminator on one of the tugs. The USS *Granville S. Hall* served as the laboratory support ship.

Phase A, conducted in May 1964 (DoD, 2004), was intended as "preliminary check of all test procedures prior to conducting the pathogenic agent phases and to obtain data to characterize diffusion in a marine environment" (DTC, 1966, p. 1). It took place in an area of open sea about 175 nautical miles southwest of Oahu, Hawaii, and included six aerial and two surface releases of BG (DTC, 1965, pp. 125, 187). For the aerial tests, the FP tracer was released at heights of 500 or 1000 feet above the sea surface, and BG was released by jet aircraft (DTC, 1965, pp. 125, 186) along each of two release lines. For the surface trials, a tug disseminated BG along an 8-mile release line (DTC, 1965, p. 187).

Phase B took place in February and March 1965, in a remote open-sea area, roughly 160 km southwest of Johnston Island. It included eight aerial releases of UL and BG together and one aerial release of UL only. For the aerial releases, jets carried two wing-mounted tanks; one tank released BG and the other UL for simultaneous dissemination along "each of one to three release lines ranging from 31 to 59 km in length" (DTC, 1965, p. 13) There were also four surface releases with both UL and BG. For each of the surface trials, a tug equipped with two E-2 multihead disseminators simultaneously disseminated UL from one head and BG from the other head along a 15-km release line (DTC, 1965, p. 13). FP was disseminated during this study to help in evaluating the meteorological conditions (DTC, 1965, pp. 6-7).

The four Phase D trials took place between March 22 and April 3, 1965, in open sea approximately 100 miles southwest of Johnston Island (DoD, 2003). A4C jets simultaneously disseminated tracer BG from one tank and OU from the other tank along several release lines (one aircraft per line). FP was also used as a tracer for this study (DTC, 1965, pp. 105, 127).

The final report includes the following statement: "Of the hundreds of personnel (Marine, Navy, Army, Air Force, and civilian) that participated in the conduct of these trials, no industrial type accidents or agent exposures resulted, thus indicating the exceptional job done in the training and execution of a test program of this magnitude by all participating personnel. It further confirmed the feasibility of using operational combat units, with a minimum amount of personnel training and experience, to deliver biological weapons on targets from remote bases throughout the world" (DTC, 1965, p. 97).

*Sources*:

DoD. 2003. *Fact sheet: Shady Grove (revised)*, version 12-2-2003. http://www.health.mil/Reference-Center/Fact-Sheets/2003/12/02/Shady-Grove-Revised (accessed September 23, 2015).

DoD. 2004 (unpublished). *SHAD test information*. Provided to the Institute of Medicine in response to an information request submitted by Susanne Stoiber, Executive Officer, Institute of Medicine, to William Winkenwerder, Assistant Secretary of Defense for Health Affairs, Department of Defense. Washington, DC.

DTC. 1965. *Test 64-4—Shady Grove (U), Final Report*. December. Redacted excerpts from cover, pp. iii-v, viii, ix, 5-7, 9, 11, 13, 22, 28, 96, 97, 105, 113, 125, 127, 185-187, 205, 206, 209, 215, 216, 221, 222. DMMC Control #2003272-0000004. Fort Douglas, UT: Deseret Test Center.

DTC. 1966. *Test 64-4 Shady Grove (U), Final Report*. June. Redacted excerpts from cover, pp. 1, 2, 7. AD 500839. Fort Douglas, UT: Deseret Test Center.

**Flower Drum II (Test 64-2)**

*November-December 1964*

The Flower Drum II test was carried out at sea in the Pacific Ocean off the coast of Oahu, Hawaii, and included 10 trials. Its purpose was "1) to investigate the effectiveness of a shipboard water washdown, both as a protective and as a decontaminant measure, against agent VX delivered from a mechanism that simulates aerial spray. 2) to obtain data and operational experience to contribute to the planning and operation of Fearless Johnny"[3] (DTC, 1965, p. 3).

The platform for the test was the US Navy covered lighter (barge) YFN-811, which was towed during the trials by the US Navy tug ATF 105. The barge was towed approximately 1 km behind the tug. A spray device on the barge disseminated the test agent, which was a dyed liquid containing approximately 90 percent VX (by weight). Radioactive "tagged VX" molecules containing the radioactive isotope phosphorus 32 were included in the agent. Bis (2 ethyl-hexyl) hydrogen phosphite was also used in this test as a simulant (DoD, 2002).

The final report describes tests of variations in timing of water washdown to determine their effectiveness in providing protection and decontamination against simulated, aerial delivery of agent VX (DTC, 1965).

The SHAD I report (IOM, 2007) noted that according to the information received from DoD, no individuals could be assigned to this test.

*Sources:*

DoD. 2002. *Fact sheet: Flower Drum, Phase II,* version 05-23-2002. http://www.health.mil/Reference-Center/Fact-Sheets/2002/05/23/Flower-Drum-Phase-II (accessed September 28, 2015).

DTC. 1965. *Test 64-2, Flower Drum (U), Phase II, Final Report.* October. Rpt. No. DTC 642105R. Redacted excerpts from cover, pp. iii, 1-3, 5, 7. Fort Douglas, UT: Deseret Test Center.

IOM (Institute of Medicine). 2007. *Long-term health effects of participation in Project SHAD (Shipboard Hazard and Defense).* Washington, DC: The National Academies Press.

## Copper Head (Test 65-1)

*January-February 1965*

The Copper Head test was carried out in the Atlantic Ocean in international waters off the coast of Newfoundland, Canada, and included 10 trials. The test ship was the USS *Power* (DD 839), and the test agent was BG, with FP used as well.

The Copper Head test was intended to determine the extent of aerosol penetration (related to particle size) into an operational ship under three conditions of readiness in a frigid environment. It was also intended to compare the travel of a biological cloud in a frigid marine environment with the travel predicted by diffusion models (DTC, 1966, p. 2).

The secondary objectives of the test included determining, in a frigid marine environment, if (a) passage of a ship through biological aerosols resulted in contamination of exterior and interior surfaces, (b) a system to spray betapropiolactone could be used under operational conditions to decontaminate an interior ship's compartment after exposure to a biological aerosol, and (c) the use of an installed exterior deck washdown system was operationally feasible. An additional aim for the test was to obtain information on the performance in the test environment of an Aero-14B-spray tank jet aircraft weapon system that was used to disseminate BG (DTC, 1966).

The final report indicates that in one of the trials, the aerosols missed the target ship (DTC, 1966). In the publicly available materials no details are provided about the use of betapropriolactone to decontaminate the ship.

[3] Fearless Johnny was another SHAD test.

*Source:*
DTC. 1966. *Test 65-1—Copper Head (U), Final Report.* March. Redacted excerpts from cover, pp. iii, iv, 2, 3, 5, 8. Rpt. No. DTC 65110BR. Fort Douglas, UT: Deseret Test Center.

### High Low (Test 65-13)

*January-February 1965*

The High Low test took place in the Pacific Ocean off the coast of San Diego. The 33 trials used methyl acetoacetate (MAA) as a simulant to investigate the potential penetration of a cloud of the nerve agent sarin into naval ships.[4] Four ship types were involved: a FRAM MK I destroyer (USS *Fechteler*, DD-870), a guided missile destroyer (USS *Berkeley*, DDG-15), a landing ship, tank (USS *Wexford County*, LST-1168), and an attack personnel transport (USS *Okanogan,* APA-220). Each ship was tested under three material readiness conditions. The simulant was disseminated from a turbine disseminator located on the bow of the test ship.

According to information provided by DoD (2004) from ship logs, the USS *Wexford County* participated in 6 trials during the period January 11-15, the USS *Okanogan* participated in 9 trials (3 at each of three material readiness conditions) between January 22 and January 26, the USS *Berkeley* participated in 9 trials (3 at each of three material readiness conditions) between February 8 and February 11, and the USS *Fechteler* participated in 9 trials (3 at each of three material readiness conditions) between February 23 and February 26.

The final test report states that "all personnel (ships' crews and civilian test personnel) were instructed in the use of the protective mask, and masks were worn by personnel directly exposed to significant quantities of MAA" (DTC, 1966, p. 9).

*Sources:*
DoD. 2003. *Fact sheet: High Low,* version 3-4-2003. http://www.health.mil/Reference-Center/Fact-Sheets/2003/03/04/High-Low (accessed October 2, 2015).
DoD. 2004 (unpublished). *SHAD test information.* Provided to the Institute of Medicine in response to an information request submitted by Susanne Stoiber, Executive Officer, Institute of Medicine, to William Winkenwerder, Assistant Secretary of Defense for Health Affairs, Department of Defense. Washington, DC.
DTC. 1966. *Test 65-13 High Low (U), Final Report.* July. Redacted excerpts from cover, pp. iii, 3, 5, 6, 9, 48, 158-173. Fort Douglas, UT: Deseret Test Center.

### Magic Sword (Test 65-4)

*May 1965*

The eight trials of the Magic Sword test were carried out on the USS *George Eastman* off the coast of Baker Island in the Pacific Ocean, and on Baker Island. The test was intended to study the feasibility of offshore release of *Aedes aegypti* mosquitoes and to obtain information on mosquito biting habits, trap technology, and operational and logistical problems associated with delivering mosquitoes to remote sites (DTC, 1966).

Uninfected mosquitoes were used for the test. Mosquitoes were released from the USS *George Eastman* shortly after dawn, and trap recoveries were checked at 3, 12, and 24 hours

---

[4] The agent–simulant relationship of MAA to sarin nerve agent had been evaluated and established in the Flower Drum Phase I test carried out in August-September 1964 (DTC 1966CH). No sarin was used in the High Low test (DoD, 2003).

after the release. Volunteers from the crew of the *George Eastman* participated in mosquito-biting trials on the 380-acre island (DTC, 1966).

In the evening after each trial, the area was sprayed with a nonpersistent insecticide using a Todd insecticide fog apparatus (TIFA) mounted on an "Army Mule" vehicle. Traps were inspected prior to the next trial to insure the effectiveness of the eradication. The final trial was conducted offshore (4.8-kilometer release). As the final step, the entire island was sprayed, using the fog apparatus and nonpersistent insecticide, and all potential breeding areas were sprayed with a 5 percent suspension of DDT in water applied by hand sprayers. Aboard the USS *George Eastman*, a combination of high heat (120°F) and insecticide were used to eradicate the mosquitoes (DTC, 1966).

*Source*:

DTC. 1966. *Test 65-4—Magic Sword (U)*. May. Redacted excerpts from pp. iii, iv, 5, 8, 9, number covered, 89, 90. Fort Douglas, UT: Deseret Test Center.

**Big Tom (Test 65-6)**

*April-June 1965*

The Big Tom test consisted of at least 19 trials carried out on the island of Oahu, Hawaii, and in the nearby waters and airspace. The test was intended to evaluate the feasibility of a biological attack on a tropical or jungle island complex and to evaluate Marine Corps doctrine and tactics for delivery of such an attack (DoD, 2003, 2004; DTC, 1967).

The final report on Big Tom describes it as being carried out in two phases (Phases A and B). In both phases, the simulant BG was released along with a tracer (DTC, 1967). In the Phase A trials, liquid BG and the tracer were disseminated from an Aero 14B spray tank mounted on a US Navy A-4 aircraft upwind from Oahu at varying heights and distances. In the Phase B trials, dry BG was released from an A/B Y45-4 spray tank mounted on a US Air Force F-105 aircraft. In both phases contractor aircraft disseminated a tracer of yellow and green zinc cadmium sulfide along the same flight path. The USS *Granville S. Hall* collected meteorological data and provided laboratory support; the ship steamed upwind of the disseminated material to avoid contamination.

The portions of the Big Tom final report that have been made public do not mention participation of a submarine or ships in the test. However, the participation of the submarine USS *Carbonero* is noted in the DoD (2003) Fact Sheet for this test, and it is also mentioned in the final report for DTC Test 68-71, Folded Arrow (DTC, 1969). That document notes that "a preliminary test, conducted in April 1965, consisted of two biological tracer (BG) trials which were designed to demonstrate the feasibility of [a submarine disseminating] system and, equally important, to determine the biological-contamination hazard to which the submarine crew would be subjected in operating the system" (DTC, 1969, pp. 4-5). The April 1965 trials, use of BPL as a "neutralizer," and participation of the USS *Carbonero* are also noted in portions of a redacted report on the test from the Navy (U.S. Naval Ordnance Test Station, 1965).

*Sources*:

DoD. 2003. *Fact sheet: Big Tom,* version 6-30-2003. http://www.health.mil/Reference-Center/Fact-Sheets/2003/06/30/Big-Tom-Update (accessed September 28, 2015).

DoD. 2004 (unpublished). *SHAD test information.* Provided to the Institute of Medicine in response to an information request submitted by Susanne Stoiber, Executive Officer, Institute of Medicine, to William Winkenwerder, Assistant Secretary of Defense for Health Affairs, Department of Defense. Washington, DC.

DTC. 1967. *Test 65-6 Big Tom (U), Final report.* January. Redacted excerpts from cover, pp. iii, 1-4, number covered, 6, 10, 14, 15, 20. Rpt. No. DTC 656126R. Fort Douglas, UT: Deseret Test Center.

DTC. 1969. *Test 68-71, Final report.* March. Redacted excerpts from cover, pp. i, iii, iv, 1, 2, 4-6, 32, 34, number covered, 43, 44, 53, 54, 56, 57. Rpt. No. DTC 6871166R. Fort Douglas, UT: Deseret Test Center.

U.S. Naval Ordnance Test Station. 1965. *Big Tom test report for Project 777.* 24 June. Redacted excerpts from cover memorandum, pp. 1, 2, 5, 7, 8. China Lake, CA: U.S. Naval Ordnance Test Station.

## Fearless Johnny (Test 65-17)

*August, September 1965*

Fearless Johnny was carried out in the Pacific Ocean southwest of Honolulu and involved 17 trials. The test agents were the nerve agent VX or its simulant, diethylphthalate (DEP), combined with 0.1 percent of fluorescent dye DF-504. The target ship was the USS *George Eastman.* Two of the light tugs served as couriers, transferring test samples between the USS *George Eastman* and support vessels. The agents were disseminated by aircraft (Navy A4-Bs) stationed at an airfield (Bonham) on the Island of Kauai. The USS *Granville S. Hall* provided laboratory support (DoD, 2004; DTC, 1966).

According to the redacted final report, the Fearless Johnny test was intended to "(1) evaluate … the magnitude of exterior and interior contamination levels under three material readiness conditions, (2) demonstrate the effectiveness of the shipboard water washdown system as a protective and decontaminant measure against VX spray, and (3) evaluate the operational impact of gross VX contamination on a U.S. Navy ship" (DTC, 1966, p. iii).

The 14 trials using the simulant DEP were carried out from August 8 to August 25, 1965, under three material readiness conditions: Yoke, Zebra, and Zebra Circle William (DTC, 1966). The three trials with VX were carried out September 10, 14, and 19 under the material readiness condition of "Zebra Circle William maximum security" (DoD, 2004).

*Sources:*

DoD. 2004 (unpublished). *SHAD test information.* Provided to the Institute of Medicine in response to an information request submitted by Susanne Stoiber, Executive Officer, Institute of Medicine, to William Winkenwerder, Assistant Secretary of Defense for Health Affairs, Department of Defense. Washington, DC.

DTC. 1966. *Test 65-17—Fearless Johnny (U), Final report.* November. Redacted excerpts from cover, pp. iii, iv, 3, 5, 7, 34. Rpt. No. DTC 6517125R. Fort Douglas, UT: Deseret Test Center.

## Purple Sage (Test 66-5)

*January-February, 1966*

Purple Sage consisted of 21 trials in which methyl acetoacetate (MAA) was used to simulate the envelopment of the test ship USS *Herbert J. Thomas* by sarin nerve agent. The test was carried out in the Pacific Ocean off the coast of San Diego, California. The test was designed to evaluate the effectiveness of the experimental Shipboard Toxicological Operational Protection System (STOPS) against attack with a gaseous chemical warfare agent in operational situations (DTC, 1967). Another objective was to evaluate the effect that wearing a protective mask (MK5 or M17) for a 4-hour period had on the operational efficiency of a ship's crew.

MAA was disseminated through a turbine disseminator located on the bow of the test ship. No information is provided about ship washdown.

*Source:*

DTC. 1967. *Test 66-5—Purple Sage (U), Final report.* January Redacted excerpts from cover, pp. iii, 5, 7. Rpt. No. DTC 6650130. Fort Douglas, UT: Deseret Test Center.

**Scarlet Sage (Test 66-6)**

*February-March 1966*

The Scarlet Sage test consisted of 19 trials that were carried out in the Pacific Ocean, off the coast of San Diego, California. The objective of this test was "to evaluate the effectiveness of the Shipboard Toxicological Operational Protective System (STOPS) against an envelopment attack of a biological aerosol" (DTC, 1967, p. iii).

For the trials, the biological aerosol simulant BG was released from a continuous point source 500 meters upwind from the target vessel, the USS *Herbert J. Thomas*, during a 10-minute period. The test included both aerial and surface release trials. Surface releases were from an E-2 BW dissemination system mounted on the AVR boat *North Island*. The data collected from aerial releases were reported as too low to read (DoD, 2004), which may mean the results were below the limit of detection of the samplers.

Other objectives for the test included determining the degree of aerosol penetration into closed but unpressurized areas of the ship; comparing the results with similar ships without STOPS, taking into account the ventilation characteristics; determining the degree of exterior and interior contamination of surfaces and evaluating the exterior water washdown system; and evaluating "the nasal pharyngeal-wash technique as a method for detecting the inhalation of biological aerosols" by exposed personnel (DTC, 1967, p. 5).

A set of data labeled "Personnel Swab Results" for 24 people shows that some of these personnel tested positive for BG after aerosol exposure, and that some of them had a positive result for a swab taken after a shower (DTC, 1967, pp. 72-74).

*Sources:*

DoD. 2004 (unpublished). *SHAD test information.* Provided to the Institute of Medicine in response to an information request submitted by Susanne Stoiber, Executive Officer, Institute of Medicine, to William Winkenwerder, Assistant Secretary of Defense for Health Affairs, Department of Defense. Washington, DC.

DTC. 1967. *Test 66-6—Scarlet Sage (U), Final report.* April. Redacted excerpts from cover, pp. iii, iv, 5, 7, 13, 14, 18, 72-74. Rpt. No. DTC 6661339. Fort Douglas, UT: Deseret Test Center.

**Half Note (Test 66-13)**

*August, September 1966*

The Half Note test took place in the open Pacific Ocean, approximately 80 miles south-southwest of Oahu. It involved at least 27 trials. The biological test agents used were *Bacillus globigii* (BG), *Serratia marcescens* (SM), and *Escherichia coli* (*EC*), with use of the tracers calcofluor (fluorescent brightener 28) and zinc cadmium sulfide (DoD, 2003). The USS *George*

*Eastman* and five light tugs (hull numbers 2080, 2082, 2085, 2086, and 2087) were target ships, with aerial dissemination of the test agents BG, SM, and EC by an A-4 aircraft and surface releases of BG from the submarine USS *Carbonero*. The USS *Granville S. Hall* provided laboratory support.

Half Note was "designed to determine biological decay rates of nonpathogenic organisms—*Escherichia coli (EC)* and *Seratia marcescens (SM)*—in a marine environment" for comparison with chamber decay rates (DTC, 1968, p. iii). For each trial, either EC or SM was released with a BG slurry. Specifically, Group A trials consisted of EC and BG, Group B of SM and BG, and Group C of EC (made through a different process than the material used in Group A) and BG. The BG also contained 1 percent phenol. For three of the Group B trials, calcofluor was added to the BG slurry (1 percent by weight). Group E used a new test concept of directly releasing the test agents over the test ship (USS *George Eastman*). FP was used as a tracer (DTC, 1968).

The DoD Fact Sheet notes the use of the USS *Carbonero* to disseminate BG in this test (DoD, 2003). The redacted version of the final report does not include this information, but the final report for the Folded Arrow test states (DTC, 1969, p. 5), "In September, 1966, the submarine weapon system disseminated a nonpathogenic biological aerosol against the downwind sampling array established for DTC Test 66-13, HALF NOTE."

The DoD Fact Sheet states that in each trial, the USS *George Eastman* and tugs would "traverse upwind attempting to remain in the aerosol cloud for several hours" (DoD, 2003, p. 1). The final report (DTC, 1968) suggests that this was done only for three of the trials (Group E).

Half Note testing included evaluating the contamination hazards to the crew of the submarine USS *Carbonero*, which was equipped with a biological weapon system. A portion of a related report (U.S. Naval Weapons Laboratory, n.d., pp. 36-37) notes that "[d]econtamination was performed in the mix area, transfer area, topside boat area, and for the nozzle." The decontamination solution was calcium hypochlorite (HTH) in water. Final decontamination of the mix area was described as a 20-minute spray of BPL, "after which the contents of the van were allowed to soak for 24 hours" (U.S. Naval Weapons Laboratory, n.d., p. 38).

*Sources:*

DoD. 2003. *Fact sheet: Half Note,* version 6-30-2003. http://www.health.mil/Reference-Center/Fact-Sheets/2002/10/09/Half-Note (accessed September 28, 2015).

DTC. 1968. *Test 66-13 (U).* March. Redacted excerpts from pp. iii, 1, 6, 7, 11, 15-17, 28, 31, 32, 40. Fort Douglas, UT: Deseret Test Center.

DTC. 1969. *Test 68-71, Final report.* March. Redacted excerpts from cover, pp. i, iii, iv, 1, 2, 4-6, 32, 34, number covered, 43, 44, 53, 54, 56, 57. Rpt. No. DTC 6871166R. Fort Douglas, UT: Deseret Test Center.

U.S. Naval Weapons Laboratory. n.d. *Project 777 contamination hazards assessment (CHA): Test report.* Redacted excerpts from cover memo, pp. 1, 36-38. China Lake, CA: U.S. Naval Ordnance Test Station.

## Folded Arrow (Test 68-71)

*April, May 1968, with additional contamination hazard assessment trials in July, 1968*

The Folded Arrow test took place near Oahu, Hawaii, using BG as a simulant for Venezuelan equine encephalitis virus (FX). It included 11 trials (DoD, 2004). The test was designed and conducted to provide "a basis upon which the U.S. Navy could recommend use of the submarine-biological disseminator weapon system for dissemination of agent FX" (DTC, 1969, p. 1). The tests were carried out after midnight to avoid destruction of the BG by sunlight.

The objective of the test "was to study over-ocean downwind travel of a biological aerosol material when disseminated from a submarine-biological system and to relate these data" to likely rates of infection from FX (DTC, 1969, p. 5). The participating ships are identified as the submarine the USS *Carbonero*, five light tugs, and the USS *Granville S. Hall* (DoD, 2003).

The six Group A trials (one was repeated because of an apparent failure) were conducted in the Pacific Ocean approximately 80 nautical miles south-southwest of Oahu. The five tugs, each of which had two sampling sites, were stationed in predetermined locations along the downwind path of the BG aerosol.

Group B and C trials used the submarine disseminator to test exposures on land. The two Group B trials, both conducted in the northern half of Oahu, were intended "to demonstrate, in terms of FX-casualty estimates, the capability of the submarine weapon system to carry out an effective biological attack against an island complex.... Sampling stations were established at 15 locations selected to best depict movement of the aerosol cloud across the island" (DTC, 1969, p. 32). The two Group C trials were intended "to study effects, in terms of estimated FX casualties, of a biological attack against a naval port facility" (DTC, 1969, p. 43). In these trials, the submarine disseminated BG along a line off-shore from Kaneohe Marine Corps Air Station on Oahu.

The Folded Arrow test also included an "elaborate evaluation program" designed to determine the contamination hazard to the submarine and crew associated with the biological dissemination system (DTC, 1969, p. 53). The evaluation "consisted primarily of aerosol and contact (swab) samples taken from numerous points inside and outside the submarine before, during, and after aerosol dissemination. Procedures to avoid contamination were developed for those shipboard personnel associated with the systems operation, especially critical for topside, posttrial decontamination exercises" (DTC, 1969, p. 53). The final report states that the contamination hazard assessment (CHA) program was also conducted "in conjunction with all previous DTC tests with the submarine system and many more times during special tests. Results demonstrated that interior contamination of the submarine is not a problem so long as prescribed procedures for the system's operation and maintenance are followed" (DTC, 1969, p. 53). The scope of the CHA was limited to the hazard "to personnel conducting the agent tank-filling operation and to shipboard personnel during operation of the weapon system. Interior and exterior assessments were made before, during, and after system operation" ( DTC, 1969, p. 54).

The Results section of the redacted final report notes the following:

> 1. Although small amounts of contamination were encountered during the 68-71 trials, it was attributed to personnel error and to ineffectiveness of Calcium Hypo-Chlorite (HTH) as a decontaminant of exterior surfaces with [sic] HTH was effective in concentrations of 6,000 to 7,500 ppm.
> 2. Additional CHA trials in July 68 (following completion of 68-71 trials) were conducted under strict tactical conditions. Beta-propiolactone (BPL), used in lieu of HTH, was found to be highly effective in decontaminating the cloud system. No trace of BPL vapor was detected within the submarine during the decontaminant tank-filling operation, or during the system decontamination phase accomplished while under way. (DTC, 1969, pp. 56-57)

*Sources:*

DoD. 2003. *Fact sheet: Folded Arrow,* version 06-30-2003. http://www.health.mil/Reference-Center/Fact-Sheets/2003/06/30/Folded-Arrow (accessed September 29, 2015).

DoD. 2004 (unpublished). *SHAD test information.* Provided to the Institute of Medicine in response to an information request submitted by Susanne Stoiber, Executive Officer, Institute of Medicine, to William Winkenwerder, Assistant Secretary of Defense for Health Affairs, Department of Defense. Washington, DC.

DTC. 1969. *Test 68-71, Final report.* March. Redacted excerpts from cover, pp. i, iii, iv, 1, 2, 4-6, 32, 34, number covered, 43, 44, 53, 54, 56, 57. Rpt. No. DTC 6871166R. DMMC Control #2003154-0000002. Fort Douglas, UT: Deseret Test Center.

**Test 69-31**

*August-September 1968*

Test 69-31 was carried out during daylight hours in the Pacific Ocean, roughly 80 nautical miles off the coast of San Diego, in the vicinity of San Clemente Island and Santa Catalina Island (DTC, 1969). It was the third and final test involving the USS *Herbert J. Thomas*, a ship that had been specially outfitted with the Shipboard Toxicological Operational Shipboard Protection System (STOPS). The 16 trials of Test 69-31 were designed to evaluate the continued effectiveness of STOPS after operational deployment.

Five trials used MAA, a simulant for sarin nerve agent, disseminated from a generator mounted on the bow of the test ship (DoD, 2002). In 11 trials, BG was disseminated from patrol boats in simulated biological warfare attacks. General quarters (GQ) was sounded before each trial began and was maintained through the completion of the sampling procedures. The final report notes, "Zone-to-zone transit within the STOPS envelope was not permitted during GQ. Following each biological trial and before securing from GQ, the ship's water-washdown system was activated for approximately 10 minutes to thoroughly flush the topside surfaces" (DTC, 1969, p. 7).

No other decontamination procedures for the test are described in the publicly available portions of the final report.

*Sources:*

DoD. 2002. *Fact sheet: DTC test 69-31,* version 10-09-2002. http://www.health.mil/Reference-Center/Fact-Sheets/2002/10/09/DTC-Test-6931 (accessed September 29, 2015).

DTC. 1969. *DTC test 69-31*, Vol I. May 29. Redacted excerpts from pp. v, vi, 1, 3, 7. Fort Douglas, UT: Deseret Test Center.

**Speckled Start (Test 68-50)**

*September-October 1968*

The 12 trials of Speckled Start were conducted at Eniwetok Atoll, Marshall Islands. The purpose of the test was "to determine the potential casualty area and associated casualty levels for the F-4/AB45Y-4/PG2 weapon system," which disseminated an aerosol over a 40-50 km downwind grid (DTC, 1969, p. 2). The grid encompassed a portion of the Eniwetok Atoll and an array of five Army light tugs.

Nine of the trials used the agent staphylococcal enterotoxin, Type B, produced by certain strains of the bacterium *Staphylococcus aureus* (DoD, 2004). A 2 percent concentration of uranine dye (sodium fluorescein) was incorporated into the agent to serve as a tracer. The trials also used BG in dried form as a tracer (DTC, 1969). An F4-E aircraft assigned to the 4533rd Tactical Test Squadron, 33rd Tactical Fighter Wing, disseminated the agent and tracers for the trials. A 91-meter tower on Ursula Islet served as the primary meteorological site for recording environmental parameters and collected data to estimate the source strength and efficiency of the weapon system. The tugs were positioned in a downwind array to determine the area covered. The USS *Granville S. Hall* was assigned to the test to provide laboratory support.

*Sources:*

DoD. 2004 (unpublished). *SHAD test information.* Provided to the Institute of Medicine in response to an information request submitted by Susanne Stoiber, Executive Officer, Institute of Medicine, to William Winkenwerder, Assistant Secretary of Defense for Health Affairs, Department of Defense. Washington, DC.

DTC. 1969. *DTC test 68-50 test report,* Vol. I. March. Redacted excerpts from pp. v, vi, 1, 2, 5. Fort Douglas, UT: Deseret Test Center.

**Test 69-10**

*May 1969*

Test 69-10 consisted of trials to determine the operational effect of an attack with a persistent, toxic, chemical agent spray on US amphibious forces while they were engaged in an amphibious assault on the beaches of Vieques Island, six miles east of Puerto Rico. The test used trioctyl phosphate (TOF) (also referred to as tri(2-ethylhexl) phosphate, or TEHP) to simulate VX nerve agent (DTC, 1969).

The test sought to assess the degradation in performance of troops wearing protective clothing, the effectiveness of existing chemical weapons, and the contamination of ships and equipment supporting the landing. The first part of the test consisted of aerial spray attacks against battalion landing team (Minus) [BLT(-)] and company-sized US Marine Corps amphibious landing forces. The second part was an aerial spray attack against the USS *Fort Snelling* (LSD-30) while it was simulating off-loading of troops for an amphibious assault. The simulant TOF was delivered by Marine A-4 aircraft carrying Aero 14 B spray tanks.

Samples were collected from exposed personnel and their clothing to determine the extent of contamination with the simulant. The performance of the troops, landing craft crews, and ship's crew in responding to the attack and subsequently operating in a simulated toxic environment was also evaluated.

*Source:*

DTC. 1969. *DTC test 69-10 (U),* Vol. I., Coordination draft, final report. Redacted excerpts from cover, pp. v, vi, 1-4, 1-5, 1-6. Fort Douglas, UT: Deseret Test Center.

**Test 69-32**

*April-June 1969*

Test 69-32 consisted of 27 trials carried out in the Pacific Ocean southwest of the Hawaiian Islands. It was conducted to evaluate the effect of sunlight on the viability of aerosolized *Serratia marcescens* and *Escherichia coli* disseminated in a temperate environment during sunrise and sunset periods (DTC, 1970).

These agents were aerosolized and released from two Aero 14B spray tanks mounted on an A4C jet aircraft. BG with 10 percent calcofluor, a fluorescent tracer suspension, was released from one tank, while either *S. marcescens* (14 trials) or *E. coli* (13 trials) was released from the other.

The five Army light tug boats were used as sampling platforms for this test. The USS *Granville S. Hall* provided laboratory support for the test and remained upwind of the dissemination.

*Source:*

DTC. 1970. *DTC test 69-32*, Vol. I. May. Redacted excerpts from cover, p. iii, v, 1-1 to 1-2, 2-1, 2-2. Fort Douglas, UT: Deseret Test Center.

**Test 70-C**

*October 1969 and 1972, February-March 1973*

DTC Test 70-C was conducted to characterize the naturally occurring airborne particulates in a marine atmosphere to provide background data needed for developing biological detectors (DoD, 2003). An additional objective was to assess the phosphorescent and fluorescent emission spectra of marine flora and fauna. No agents or simulants were used.

According to the DoD Fact Sheet, testing was conducted twice. In October 1972 the USNS *Samuel Phillips Lee* served as the sampling platform in an area 50-65 miles off the coast of San Diego. In 1973 the USNS *Silas Bent* collected samples as it traveled from San Diego to Rodman Naval Station, Balboa, Canal Zone.

Weekly status reports from the USS *Granville S. Hall* indicate that in October 1969 it was also carrying out sampling in support of test 70-C (Department of the Navy, 1969a,b).

*Sources:*

Department of the Navy. 1969a. Weekly status report for period ending 24 October 1969. 28 Oct.

Department of the Navy. 1969b. Weekly status report for period ending 31 October 1969. 3 Nov.

DoD. *2003. Fact sheet: DTC Test 70-C,* version 6-30-2003. http://www.health.mil/Reference-Center/Fact-Sheets/2003/06/30/DTC-Test-70-C (accessed September 29, 2015).

# 3

# Data and Methods for the SHAD II Study

The Shipboard Hazard and Defense (SHAD) II study was conducted to respond to continued concerns that Project SHAD veterans may be experiencing increased long-term health effects or mortality that are associated with their participation in SHAD tests during the 1960s. This chapter describes the design of the SHAD II study and reviews the details of the study population, the measures of exposure and health outcomes, and the approach to the analysis. It also notes some of the challenges in trying to study the experience of these veterans and limitations in the data available for the study and describes important differences between the SHAD I and SHAD II studies. A discussion of the technical details of the analytic methods chosen for the SHAD II study and their application is provided in Appendix D.

## NEW APPROACHES IN SHAD II

The SHAD I study (IOM, 2007) constituted a major effort to identify veterans who participated in the SHAD tests, select an appropriate comparison population, define indicators of exposure, and assess a range of health outcomes. The SHAD II study presented an opportunity to build on this previous work. For SHAD II, the committee adopted new approaches in three areas: (1) proposing a set of literature-based a priori hypotheses about health outcomes that might be expected to be associated with exposure to certain substances used in the SHAD tests; (2) attempting to refine the assessment of individuals' potential exposures to specific substances; and (3) obtaining information about health outcomes for members of the study population from records of health care services received between 1999 and 2011, as reflected in Medicare databases of the Centers for Medicare & Medicaid Services (CMS) and from 1997 through 2011 from the Department of Veterans Affairs (VA) health services.

### Hypotheses on Health Outcomes

The SHAD I study commissioned a set of papers that summarized the literature on the physical, chemical, and toxicological properties of the test substances and on the presence or absence of health effects of exposures of various types (e.g., inhalation, ingestion).[1] These papers provided essential background information for the analyses that compared a broad range of health outcomes among SHAD participants with those among the comparison population.

For SHAD II, the committee also sought to frame hypotheses it could test regarding SHAD exposures and outcomes. To that end, committee members reviewed the commissioned papers as well as reports published between January 2000 and January 2012 that considered the potential health effects of exposure to the substances used in the SHAD tests. For each of the substances, the Institute of Medicine (IOM) research librarian carried out targeted searches of Medline, Toxline, Embase, the Science Citation Index within the Web of Science, Chemical Carcinogenesis Research Information System (CCRIS), Hazardous Substances Data Bank (HSDB), and Integrated Risk Information System (IRIS). These searches used the substance's typical name(s) and its Chemical Abstracts Service (CAS) registry number, if appropriate. The searches were designed to identify literature evaluating the safety or potential long-term effects of exposure to the substances from studies in vitro, in animals, or in humans. Papers reporting use of the substances in laboratory procedures without evaluation of health effects were not considered relevant, nor were papers in which the substance was not the focus of the study.

On the basis of these reviews, the committee formulated hypotheses that certain adverse outcomes might be more likely for SHAD participants in tests that used any of six particular substances (see Table 3-1): *Coxiella burnetii* (*C. burnetii*), *Escherichia coli* (*E. coli*), Staphylococcal enterotoxin type B (SEB), sarin, betapropiolactone, and zinc cadmium sulfide. These hypotheses were seen as an opportunity to focus a portion of the analysis in a way that was not attempted in the IOM's previous SHAD study, and were not intended as a weight-of-evidence review to conclusively attribute them to the exposures. The analysis of health outcomes considered morbidity, represented by record of an inpatient or outpatient diagnosis for any of the potentially associated conditions. For those conditions that might be an underlying cause of death, the analysis also included consideration of mortality. A summary of the reviews and a list of the papers that were examined appear in Appendix C.

**Refining Exposure Metrics**

Ideally, a study of the potential health effects of an exposure would be able to make use of a quantitative measurement of the dose received by each member of the study population to look for evidence of increasing risks for given adverse health outcomes with increasing doses of a given agent. Often, however, levels of exposure must be assessed less directly. When that is necessary, levels may be defined qualitatively (e.g., high, medium, low) and may be based on indirect markers of exposure such as time spent in a particular job assignment.

Because the SHAD tests were generally designed to assess physical penetration of ship spaces by the test substances, or the effectiveness of protective gear, information on human exposure was not systematically collected. For the SHAD I study, an individual's exposure was defined most broadly as any participation in any SHAD test. Additional analyses grouped individuals based on the substances used in the tests in which they had participated. Four of these

---

[1] These papers were prepared in 2004 and are available at http://iom.nationalacademies.org/reports/2007/long-term-health-effects-of-participation-in-project-shad-shipboard-hazard-and-defense.aspx.

**TABLE 3-1** Hypotheses to Be Tested Concerning Certain Substances Used in SHAD Testing and Adverse Health Outcomes

| Substance | Use in SHAD Test | Health Outcome Hypothesized |
| --- | --- | --- |
| *Coxiella burnetii* | Biological agent | Chronic hepatitis<br>Endocarditis<br>Fatigue syndrome<br>Osteomyelitis<br>Vascular infection |
| *Escherichia coli* | Biological simulant | Irritable bowel syndrome |
| Staphylococcal enterotoxin type B[a] | Biological agent | Asthma<br>Graves' disease<br>Multiple sclerosis<br>Rheumatoid arthritis |
| Sarin | Chemical agent | Neurological effects (central nervous system)<br>Neurological effects (peripheral nervous system)<br>Neurological effects (hearing loss)<br>Psychological symptoms |
| Betapropiolactone | Decontaminant | Cancer (any type) |
| Zinc cadmium sulfide | Tracer | Chronic kidney disease<br>Lung cancer |

[a] Because the individuals who served on the vessels involved in testing staphylococcal enterotoxin type B were not identified, the committee could not test the hypotheses generated for this agent.

exposure groups were defined: Group A for simulants *Bacillus globigii* (BG) or methylacetoacetate (MAA) only; Group B for simulant trioctyl phosphate (TOF) only; Group C for any active nerve or biological agent (with or without simulant exposure); and Group D for other substances or combinations of substances, excluding any active agents. These groups are described further in the SHAD I report (IOM, 2007).

For the SHAD II study, the committee sought to refine the representation of exposure within the limits of the information available. Although the more desirable forms of exposure data were still not available, the committee took advantage of other information to characterize potential variations in exposure among the SHAD veterans in ways that were not attempted in the SHAD I study. One step was to make use of information about the number of tests, and the number of trials within each test, in which a SHAD veteran was a participant. This information made it possible to estimate the number of potential exposures to a test substance each participant may have received. The committee also chose to group exposures to biological agents separately from exposures to chemicals.

The formulation and application of these exposure indicators in the SHAD II analysis are discussed further in Appendix D.

### Obtaining Information About Health Outcomes

Identifying health outcomes, which include deaths and illnesses, among the SHAD participants and the comparison population of military veterans was a crucial part of both the SHAD I and SHAD II studies.

*Deaths (Mortality)*

Both studies relied on the National Death Index (NDI) as a source of information on causes of death for men who died in 1979 or subsequently. The NDI, which is operated by the National Center for Health Statistics, maintains a compilation of information from states' death certificates issued from 1979 forward (NCHS, 2015), and can provide data on cause of death. Records for deaths that occurred before 1979 are held by individual states. For the SHAD II study, an effort was made to obtain information on the causes of as many of these pre-1979 deaths as possible, a step that was not feasible for the SHAD I study.

*Illnesses (Morbidity)*

The SHAD I and SHAD II studies took fundamentally different approaches to determining the health status of the surviving members of the study population. For SHAD I, an extensive survey was used to collect self-reported information on physical and mental health status, health history, and related information such as smoking history. SHAD II used records of from Medicare and VA of health care received by members of the study population. The alternate approach was used to obtain data that was more representative of the entire study population than that used in SHAD I. The response rate for the SHAD I survey was 61 percent for SHAD participants and 47 percent for the comparison population.

While surveys have the advantages of using a single framework for collecting information and of obtaining information about the respondents' behaviors, experiences, and perceptions that are not consistently captured in medical records, they are vulnerable to biases related to self-reports (e.g., flawed recall and nonresponse). Records generated in conjunction with the delivery of health care services offer diagnostic information produced over many years and with the benefit of clinical expertise. The records of health care services used in the SHAD II study already exist in electronic form and do not vary by exposure status (i.e., participation in SHAD or not) or depend on the accuracy or completeness of a respondent's recall or response. This approach was not suitable at the time of the SHAD I study, when only 18 percent of the study population were age 65 or older and age-eligible for Medicare services. At the time the SHAD II study follow up concluded, 83 percent of the surviving members of the study population were age-eligible for Medicare services

## STUDY DESIGN

As in SHAD I, the SHAD II study was a retrospective cohort design (Hulley et al., 2013). With this approach, the exposure(s) of interest and the recording of health outcomes all occurred in the past. The data were collected for purposes other than the study, such as in electronic clinical or administrative databases. The study was conducted with the oversight and approval of the National Academy of Sciences, Engineering, and Medicine Committee to Review Studies on Human Subjects.

All cohort studies, including the SHAD studies, face the challenge of ensuring the comparability of the exposed group to the comparison population and controlling for factors that could lead to a spurious presence or absence of an association between the exposure and health effect. The SHAD I study sought to maximize the comparability of the comparison group by selecting military personnel from comparable ships or Marine Corps units that were serving at the same time as the units that participated in the SHAD tests. Use of this comparison population counters the concerns that might be anticipated if the SHAD participants were compared to a group of civilians or military personnel who were not deployed. The SHAD II study used the same comparison population.

A major assumption in the selection of the comparison group is that the two groups are at similar risk for other potentially health-altering exposures, including combat duty in Vietnam, behaviors known to influence health outcomes (e.g., alcohol and tobacco use), and post-SHAD employment. The SHAD I health survey found that similar percentages of the SHAD and the comparison respondents had ever smoked cigarettes (79.1 percent and 82.5 percent, respectively) or currently drank alcohol (58.2 percent and 57.1 percent, respectively). Similarly, data from the Veterans Benefits Administration (VBA) showed that 17.4 percent of SHAD participants and 18.4 percent of the comparison group had been identified as having service in Vietnam.[2]

## STUDY POPULATION

### Identifying SHAD Participants

For the first SHAD study, the Department of Defense (DoD) assembled an initial roster of Project SHAD participants and updated the roster as new information was gathered. The IOM staff independently reviewed the quarterly unit rosters (BuPers Report 1080-14) as well as the daily personnel diaries for each ship in each test to compile lists of personnel present on the vessels involved in Project SHAD tests. When the IOM identified personnel who were not on the DoD lists, these names were provided to DoD for review and validation. The IOM kept in its study only those men that DoD could validate as SHAD participants and excluded those that DoD could not validate (IOM, 2007, p. 16). On the advice of the SHAD I advisory committee, the IOM staff undertook additional outreach efforts to inform the veteran community of the study and encourage those who might have been SHAD participants to contact DoD to be included in the study. No more than two study participants were added through these efforts.

The statement of task for the SHAD II study stipulated that the same population of SHAD participants and their comparison group that had been collected and validated for the SHAD I study was to be used in the SHAD II study. The IOM therefore did not repeat its independent review of personnel diaries and quarterly reports. However, the IOM did request and receive from DoD an updated listing of SHAD participants (as of December 2012) and reviewed it to ensure that any SHAD participants who had been newly identified since the completion of the SHAD I study were not missed. The IOM's review of the updated DoD listing resulted in the addition of nine men to the population of SHAD participants. These men were participants in nine different SHAD tests.

For an individual to be considered eligible for inclusion in the SHAD I study, it was necessary to have information sufficient to uniquely identify him for purposes of contact for the survey. For the SHAD II study, 19 men were excluded because the available information (name or service number) was insufficient to determine their social security numbers, the identifier by which information was extracted from records on vital status and health care services received.

---

[2] These data are for veterans who have filed a disability claim and were identified by VBA as having had Vietnam service. Vietnam service is defined as duty or visitation within the country of South Vietnam, including Navy veterans who entered inland waterways on ships, went ashore from offshore ships, or served only aboard offshore ships and never went ashore or entered inland waterways (Personal communication, J. Sampsel, Veterans Benefits Administration, March 12, 2014).

An additional 42 men were found to be ineligible because they were participants in (or from comparison units for) Project 112 tests that were not part of SHAD testing. Also, despite the data validation efforts by DoD and the IOM, three men were excluded because they had dates of death that preceded the dates of the SHAD tests in which they were supposed to have participated. An additional six men whose records indicated that they were dead but for whom dates of death were missing were included in the study population, but they could not be included in the survival analysis described in Chapter 4.

### SHAD Comparison Group

As described in greater detail in the report on the SHAD I study (IOM, 2007), the SHAD comparison population was drawn from two sources. Each ship in a SHAD test was matched, to the extent possible, with a ship of a similar class, crew complement, operating area, and home port at the time of the SHAD test. For Marine Corps units, the comparison groups were selected to be similar units in operation at the same time as the SHAD test; where possible the identical unit in a parallel battalion or division was selected. The list of comparison units is provided in Appendix E.

Once the comparison ships or units were selected, the individuals serving on the ships or with those Marine Corps units were identified using a process similar to that used for the participant ships. Quarterly reports were obtained for the time period of the test and the name, military service number, and rate or job title were recorded for each person in the unit at the corresponding time. In this manner, 6,753 individuals (including 6,137 Navy, 614 Marines) were identified to serve as the comparison population for the study of the 5,868 service members (including 5,066 Navy, and 750 Marines) identified as participants in the SHAD testing.

One exception to this process was for the Navy service members who served on the five light tug boats that participated in the SHAD testing. These tugs were used to set up sampling arrays in the open ocean for the tests of active biological agents and simulants, as well as in one known instance, they were used as couriers of samples. The tugs were originally built for the Army, but were specially modified with small laboratory spaces for use as sampling stations for the SHAD testing. No comparable vessels were part of the regular Navy fleet, and as a result no comparison ships and crews could be identified. Moreover, crew records for the tugs were not maintained in the same fashion as for the other ships. The only test for which a list that identifies men who served on the tugs (9-12 men per vessel) is available is Shady Grove. The list includes members of the Project SHAD technical staff who were detailed as crew members of the five light tugs and to the laboratory ship, the USS *Granville S. Hall*. The choice of a comparison group for the personnel from the tugs and Project SHAD technical staff is discussed in Appendix D.

## ASSESSING EXPOSURE

The SHAD tests involved at least 19 different vessels and 7 Marine Corps units in 21 tests that used at least 16 different test substances (alone or in combination) over a period of 7 years. Each test included multiple trials, ranging from as few as five trials (Test 69-10) to as many as 31 (Flower Drum I). The units that participated and the substances that were used could vary from trial to trial within a test. Some ships were involved in only one test whereas others participated in multiple tests. Ships that participated in multiple tests had changes in crew members from test to test. Approximately 69 percent of the SHAD participants (4,050 men) were in only one test. The remainder participated in from two to seven tests. Because the nature of the tests varied widely, the nature of SHAD veterans' potential exposures also vary.

Information about the substances used in the SHAD tests—active agents, simulants, tracers, and decontaminants—was available to the committee from three sources. The fact sheets for each Project SHAD test that DoD prepared and posted online[3] give summary information about the substances used in the tests, the units involved, and the range of test dates. Additional detail about many of the tests and the substances used was available to the committee from declassified portions of the final reports and other documents prepared by the Deseret Test Center at the time the tests were being conducted. In addition, information on the dates of each test's trials and test substances was compiled by DoD in 2004 during its efforts to identify and declassify information sought for the IOM SHAD I study.

Environmental concentrations of test substances are frequently used as alternative indicators of potential human doses. Although environmental readings were collected in many SHAD tests, the data remain classified and were not available to the committee. To characterize exposures that SHAD participants may have received to the substances used in the various tests, the committee used multiple approaches. First, a strictly qualitative approach grouped SHAD participants on the basis of the substances used in the tests in which they participated. Second, combining information on the substances used in SHAD tests with the number of exposure opportunities represented by number of trials within each test also made it possible to group participants on the basis of higher and lower levels of presumed exposure to certain substances.

### Qualitative Exposure Groups Related to Test Substances

Some SHAD tests made use of a single substance, but many used a combination of substances (e.g., a simulant and a tracer). As a result many of the test participants were exposed to multiple substances. For the SHAD II study, the committee created substance-specific exposure groups for the six substances for which hypotheses regarding health outcomes were formulated, The committee also created three broad exposure groups based on the substances used in the SHAD tests: (1) any biological substance; (2) any chemical substance, except trioctyl phosphate (TOF); and (3) any decontaminant. This approach was used to examine the potential for a broad category of test substances to be associated with adverse health outcomes within a group with a variety of specific exposure experiences. Exposure groups 1, 2, and 3 are not mutually exclusive; a SHAD test participant might be included in any or all of them.

The committee also carried out analyses of three groups with distinctive aspects of their exposures: (1) the crew of the USS *George Eastman*, a specially outfitted ship involved in multiple tests including some with live agents; (2) members of the Project SHAD technical staff who were identified in a roster from January 1965, with additional persons with service on the light tugs; and (3) participants in Test 69-10 who received unique exposure to TOF. The membership of these special groups was largely mutually exclusive. The potential exposures to these groups are listed in Box 3-1.

---

[3] See http://www.health.mil/Military-Health-Topics/Health-Readiness/Environmental-Exposures/Project-112-SHAD/Fact-Sheets (accessed October 15, 2015).

**BOX 3-1**
**Potential Exposures to Subgroups Special Interest**

*Biological Substances*
- *Bacillus globigii* (BG)
- *Bacillus globigii* with phenol
- *Coxiella burnetii*
- *Escherichia coli* (*E. coli*)
- *Pasteurella tularensis* (*Francisella tularensis*)
- *Serratia marcescens* (SM)
- Staphylococcal enterotoxin type B (SEB)

*Chemical Substances (except TOF)*
- Calcofluor
- Diethylphthlate
- Diethylphthlate mixed with 0.1 percent of fluorescent dye DF-504
- Insecticide
- Methyl acetoacetate (MAA)
- Sarin
- Sulfur dioxide
- Uranine (sodium fluorescein)
- VX
- Zinc cadmium sulfide

*Decontaminants*
- Betapropiolactone
- Calcium hypochlorite
- Heat of 120°F
- Insecticide

*Trioctyl phosphate (TOF)*
- Also known as tris(2-ethylhexyl) phosphate (TEHP)

*USS* George Eastman *Crew*
- *Bacillus globigii* (BG)
- *Bacillus globigii with* phenol
- Betapropiolactone
- Calcium hypochlorite
- Calcofluor
- *Coxiella burnetii*
- Diethylphthlate
- *Escherichia coli* (*E. coli*)
- Heat of 120°F
- Insecticide
- Methyl acetoacetate (MAA)
- *Pasteurella tularensis* (*Francisella tularensis*)
- Sarin
- *Serratia marcescens* (SM)
- Sulfur dioxide
- VX
- Zinc cadmium sulfide

*Light Tugs and Project SHAD Technical Staff on USS* Granville S. Hall
- *Bacillus globigii* (BG)
- *Bacillus globigii*/phenol
- Betapropiolactone
- Calcium hypochlorite
- Calcofluor
- *Escherichia coli* (*E. coli*)
- *Serratia marcescens* (SM)
- Staphylococcal enterotoxin type B (SEB)
- Sulfur dioxide
- Uranine (sodium fluorescein)
- Zinc cadmium sulfide
- (also reported, ethylene oxide)

The comparison group for each of these six exposure groups was determined on the basis of the tests in which the exposures occurred, the units in the test that received the specified exposure, and the designated comparison unit for that test. The selection of these comparison groups is described further in Appendix D.

Special consideration was also given to the crew of the USS *Granville S. Hall*, which served as the laboratory ship for many of the SHAD tests. Because of its role, care was taken to keep the ship upwind from the tests specifically to avoid exposure to the test substances. The ship's regular crew was supplemented by identified members of the Project SHAD technical staff. Regular crew other than the laboratory staff were not permitted in the laboratory area or to handle samples (Personal communication, J. Alderson, U.S. Navy Reserve (Ret.), January 2012).

For overall analyses, the committee included all *Granville S. Hall* crew members as part of the Project SHAD study population. For analyses that addressed specific forms of exposure, the Project SHAD technical staff was considered as potentially exposed and the members of the regular crew were excluded as unexposed.

## Accounting for Trials as Well as Tests

Through a detailed review of the available documentation on each test, the study staff compiled information on the dates of the trials in each test, the test substances used for each trial, the equipment and patterns used to disperse test substances, and the ships or other units participating in the trial. Summaries of this information are provided in the annex to Chapter 2. The data compiled by the study staff were tabulated to arrive at cumulative numbers of exposure events for each of the test substances for each individual identified as being present during the test period. Presence during a trial was established from information the IOM staff collected from the Navy quarterly unit rosters and a review of the daily personnel diaries for each ship, which noted individuals who came on or left the ship each day. Similarly, information from monthly personnel rosters for Marines was augmented with company diaries regarding the movement of individuals into and out of units during the test trials (IOM, 2007). Committee members reviewed the source materials and the compiled information on trial exposures as well as the procedures used to tabulate the exposure hits received by each member of the group of test participants.

"Exposure" for each SHAD participant was represented by the number of trials within each test and the number of potential exposure opportunities for a given test substance within each trial.[4] Each exposure opportunity was counted. For example, if a sailor were present on the USS *Navarro* for all of the nine trials of the Autumn Gold test and for the three trials the *Navarro* participated in during the Eager Belle II test, he would be considered to have 12 exposures (9 + 3 = 12) to BG. If he was on the ship for the three Eager Belle II trials and for only five trials during the Autumn Gold test, he would have a total of 8 exposures (5 + 3 = 8), and so on. Because some trials included release of more than one sprayed "line" of a test substance, each line was considered to constitute an exposure opportunity and counted as an additional exposure. This approach was used to generate a count of potential exposures to each separate test substance for each individual.

In addition to tallying the number of exposure opportunities individuals had for a test substance, the committee considered their distribution among the SHAD participants. For some substances, the exposed participants had all similar numbers of exposure opportunities, but for others the number of potential exposures varied widely. Where the size of the exposed group and the variation in the number of potential exposures were considered sufficient, the committee established subgroups to reflect the range of exposure experience (e.g., low, medium, high) among the SHAD participants. Appendix D includes a description of the process used to evaluate the distribution of hits and determine the exposure subgroups.

---

[4] For the purposes of this report, "test substance" refers to any of the active agents, simulants, tracers, and decontaminants reported by DoD to have been used in each given test.

### Classified Data Concerning Exposure

As previously noted, information from many documents (e.g., test plans, final reports) from the Project SHAD tests remains classified and was not available to the committee for its work. Although many documents are automatically declassified after 25 years, the records on SHAD concern testing of chemical and biological agents and the automatic declassification rules do not apply (Personal communication, M. Kilpatrick, Department of Defense, January 19, 2012). In its 2000-2003 investigation of Project 112/SHAD, DoD committed to declassifying "medically relevant" information, but it did not include information such as nozzle size or concentrations of test agents sprayed out of concern that the information on delivery concentration could be calculated. Many of the SHAD-related DoD documents, including the declassified materials, that the committee had access to are identified in the Chapter 2 annex. All of the materials available to the committee are also publicly available.[5]

## HEALTH OUTCOMES

Health outcomes were evaluated for this study using data on mortality (timing and underlying cause of death) and morbidity (diagnoses received from inpatient and outpatient care).

### Mortality

Mortality follow up for SHAD participants began at the date of their first test exposure, and ended on the date of death or December 31, 2011, whichever came first. For the members of the comparison group, mortality follow up began on the first day of the test for which their vessel or unit was selected as a comparison unit. As of the end of follow up for the SHAD I study (December 31, 2004), 22 percent of SHAD veterans and 21 percent of the comparison population had been identified as deceased (IOM, 2007). The vital status of the remaining members of the study population—whether they were known to be dead or presumed alive on December 31, 2011—was established for the current study using VBA records and information available through Lexis/Nexis.

VBA gathers reports of veterans' deaths through notifications from Veterans Health Administration (VHA) facilities, family members applying for death benefits, or VA's National Cemetery Administration. It also obtains information through an automated match with the Social Security Administration (SSA) Death Master File. Historically, ascertainment of deaths through the VA benefits system has been found to be nearly complete. Lexis/Nexis was another source of vital status information. A comparison of the SHAD study population with the VBA records and Lexis/Nexis led to ascertainment of 1,347 new deaths since the final ascertainment for the SHAD I study.

---

[5] The declassified portions of the SHAD II reports are publicly available from the DoD Freedom of Information Act (FOIA) Reading Room at http://www.dod.mil/pubs/foi/readingRoom.html (accessed November 16, 2015). Additional information is available through the Public Access Records Office of the National Academies of Sciences, Engineering, and Medicine.

## Cause of Death

Information on underlying cause of death for members of the study population was obtained in four ways: (1) from the search of the National Death Index (NDI) Plus database that was conducted for SHAD I; (2) from a search of the VA/DoD records on cause of death for veterans, which also draws on NDI Plus; (3) from a direct search of NDI Plus requested by the IOM staff; and (4) from death certificates obtained from state vital records offices for men who died before 1979. Overall, a cause of death was ascertained for 91 percent of the men determined to be deceased by the end of study follow up, December 31, 2011. The cause of death was not successfully obtained for the remaining 9 percent of deceased men. In some cases the cause of death was not obtained because there was not a good match with the NDI Plus database.

For the 162 SHAD participants and 206 members of the comparison population who died before 1979, identifying causes of death required determining the state in which the person died and submitting a request to the state's vital records office for a copy of the death certificate. Each state has its own procedures and requirements for processing such requests. Because place of death is not reliably recorded in the records on the members of the study population from VA and DoD, the IOM staff supplemented information on residence and claims processing from VA and DoD records with searches of electronic death indexes maintained by some states and of other online genealogic resources. Requests for death certificates were submitted to 34 states, the District of Columbia, and the Philippines, resulting in the receipt of 184 death certificates from 28 states. Other online sources produced information on an additional 14 early deaths among the SHAD study population.

For deaths that occurred before January 1, 1979, cause of death may be missing because place of death could not be identified and the death certificate could not be requested; a requested death certificate was not located by the state vital records office; or it was not possible to successfully meet a state's requirements for access to vital records. Additional details regarding steps used to ascertain cause of death are provided in Appendix D.

## Morbidity

The SHAD II study assessed morbidity through records collected into automated databases as a byproduct of medical care received through VA (1997-2011) or under the auspices of Medicare billing (1999-2011). After leaving military service, some veterans receive medical care from VA facilities, many receive care from clinicians and facilities in the community, and some may receive care from both sources. On reaching age 65, almost all veterans become eligible for Medicare, but some may continue to receive some or all of their care through the VA or private insurance. The majority of US veterans have private health insurance or are eligible for Medicare and typically receive their care from sources outside VA (Shen et al., 2003; VA, n.d.-a; Westat, 2010).

### *VA Inpatient and Outpatient Visits*

For veterans who use the VA health care system, diagnostic data are available from automated records for inpatient and outpatient medical encounters from October 1999 to the present (VA, n.d.-b). Records through December 31, 2011, were used for the study. In some cases, records of VA health care provided to those in the study population were available from late 1997, and these were used where available. Eligibility for VA health services is generally based on a combination of criteria for minimum length of active duty service and the terms of discharge from military service. Additional criteria concerning a veteran's health status, military service, and income level are used to determine eligibility for one of eight priority groups, which are used to manage demand for VA health care services. Veterans classified as at least 50 percent disabled for a service-connected condition qualify for the highest priority.

For this study, the committee drew on information available from multiple VHA datasets, including Inpatient Encounters (IE), Bed section acute care dataset (PB), Main acute care dataset (PM), Procedure acute care dataset (PP), Surgery acute care dataset (PS), and Event dataset (SE). The files captured overlapping information on inpatient and outpatient encounters among those who use VHA health care services.

*Medicare Data*

Medicare is a federal health insurance program for people age 65 and older and certain persons who are younger and meet Social Security Administration requirements for disability. Once people are enrolled in Medicare, electronic records (i.e., claims) for each of their medical encounters that are processed by the Centers for Medicare & Medicaid Services (CMS) are retained. These records include information about the date of care, the reasons (diagnosis), and the type of care received. Records of these medical care claims are potentially available for use in research upon approval of investigators' ability to protect the privacy of study subjects. Medicare data are widely used for studies of health care including studies of effectiveness, access to care, disease incidence, and outcomes of care. Estimates suggest that approximately 96 percent of those who are eligible on the basis of age are covered by Medicare (EBRI, 2003).

Medicare enrollment information is provided in the Master Beneficiary Summary File (formerly the Denominator File). This file contains on an annual basis information about Medicare enrollment status and eligible benefits as well as demographic data and information about mortality. Medicare files on health care use are divided by the type of service provided. The Medicare Provider Analysis and Review (MedPAR) file contains information about hospital stays. The Outpatient and Carrier files contain information about services provided in non-inpatient facilities and care by physicians.

There are important limitations of Medicare data that must be acknowledged. First, the Medicare data do not include information about health care that is provided outside of the Medicare program. Second, the data do not include information about care provided by Medicare Managed Care enrollees. Medicare data contain information only about conditions for which diagnoses have been recorded as part of a health care claim. Some conditions that could have been (or should have been) diagnosed are not recorded. For example, dementia has consistently been shown to be under-recognized in clinical settings (e.g., Mitchell et al., 2011), and therefore is also missing from the Medicare data. Finally, Medicare records inconsistently capture information about health behaviors or risk factors such as tobacco use and obesity. Many of these limitations also apply to VHA data.

## DATA PROCESSING AND ANALYSIS

To meet VA requirements for the protection of the personally identifiable data that were the foundation for the study, it was necessary for all the data to be stored and used within the VA's information technology system, known as VINCI (VA Informatics and Computing

Infrastructure).[6] Once data from separate sources were matched, analysis files were created using case numbers without name and social security number. Data management was handled through Structure Query Language. All analyses were performed using Statistical Analysis System (SAS) or R software. The principal analyses were Kaplan-Meier survival analyses and Cox proportional hazards regression analyses for mortality, and logistic regression, Fisher's exact tests, and Wilcoxon rank-sum tests for indicators of morbidity, including median hospital days.

The data were cleaned and prepared by members of the study staff, and analyses were carried out by a consultant to the study. For each analysis undertaken, counts and simpler analyses such as percentages were confirmed by study staff using Microsoft Access. The committee determined the analyses to be performed and reviewed the results; committee members did not have access to the individual level data on health outcomes or the VINCI system where the analyses were run. Some statistical analyses that did not require access to the individual level data were carried out by a committee member. At several steps in the planning and performance of the analyses, a committee member reviewed elements of the SAS code used to ensure their appropriateness. The entire committee regularly reviewed results of the analyses and checked for consistency and interpretability. When questions arose, the committee proposed validation and alternative analyses.

Under the requirements governing use of data from CMS and in order to apply a consistent approach to all health outcome data, cell counts of 10 or less were reported only as ≤10. In situations where a simple calculation could permit reconstruction of a small cell size, the table shows NR, for not reported. The committee reported confidence intervals without the point estimates for results of analyses for which it was feasible to reconstruct a small cell size. Additional detail about analytical approaches is provided in Chapters 4 and 5 and Appendix D.

## REFERENCES

EBRI (Employee Benefit Research Institute). 2003. *Health insurance and the elderly*. Facts from EBRI. Washington, DC: EBRI. http://www.ebri.org/pdf/publications/facts/0803fact.pdf (accessed October 27, 2015).

Hulley, S. B., S. R. Cummings, W. S. Browner, D. G. Grady, and T. B. Newman. 2013. *Designing clinical research*. Philadelphia, PA: Lippincott Williams & Wilkins.

IOM (Institute of Medicine). 2007. *Long-term health effects of participation in Project SHAD (Shipboard Hazard and Defense)*. Washington, DC: The National Academies Press.

Mitchell, A. J., N. Meader, and M. Pentzek. 2011. Clinical recognition of dementia and cognitive impairment in primary care: A meta-analysis of physician accuracy. *Acta Psychiatrica Scandinavica* 124:165-183.

NCHS (National Center for Health Statistics). 2015. *National Death Index*. http://www.cdc.gov/nchs/ndi.htm (accessed October 13, 2015).

Rothman, K. J., S. Greenland, and T. L. Lash. 2008. *Modern epidemiology*, 3rd ed. Philadelphia, PA: Lippincott Williams & Wilkins.

Shen, Y., A. Hendricks, S. Zhang, and L. E. Kazis. 2003. VHA enrollees' health care coverage and use of care. *Medical Care Research Review* 60:253-267.

---

[6] Data files and programs used in this analysis will be stored on VINCI following completion of this study to the extent permitted by the respective data use agreements under which the IOM was given access to the data and subject to the conditions of the agreement with VA regarding use of its VINCI system. It is anticipated VA will retain the data and programs for at least 1 year.

VA (Department of Veterans Affairs). n.d.-a. *2001 national survey of veterans: Final report.* http://www.va.gov/VETDATA/docs/SurveysAndStudies/NSV_Final_Report.pdf (accessed October 27, 2015).

VA. n.d.-b. *Corporate data warehouse: VA informatics and computing infrastructure.* http://www.hsrd.research.va.gov/for_researchers/vinci/cdw.cfm (accessed October 27, 2015).

Westat. 2010. *National survey of veterans, active duty service members, demobilized National Guard and reserve members, family members, and surviving spouses*. Final Report. Rockville, MD: Westat. http://www.va.gov/SURVIVORS/docs/NVSSurveyFinalWeightedReport.pdf (accessed September 24, 2015).

# 4

# The Mortality Experience of SHAD Veterans

This chapter begins with a description of essential characteristics of the study population. It goes on to present the results of the committee's analyses to assess whether Project SHAD (Shipboard Hazard and Defense) veterans have experienced greater mortality than the veterans in the comparison group who served at a similar time and in similar units. Results of the analysis of morbidity data are presented in Chapter 5. A discussion of the committee's interpretation of the results is provided in Chapter 6.

## CHARACTERISTICS OF THE STUDY POPULATION

The population for this study was made up of 5,868 Project SHAD participants and 6,753 other veterans who served as a comparison group. All members of the study population were men. Chapter 3 provides details on the development of this study population. Some of the basic characteristics of the study population are shown in Table 4-1.

Overall, the SHAD participants and the comparison population are similar in their age profiles. By the end of the study follow-up period, 15 to 16 percent of the two groups remained too young (less than age 65) to qualify for Medicare enrollment. At the time of the SHAD I study, nearly 70 percent of the study population had not yet reached age 65. Among those with known race, the proportions of white and non-white service members were similar in the two groups. The SHAD participant and comparison groups are also broadly similar in terms of branches of service and rank. Substantial majorities of both groups served in the Navy and were enlisted personnel rather than officers.

Because the SHAD tests occurred during the period of the Vietnam War, the committee was concerned that service in Vietnam or presumed exposure to Agent Orange among members of the study population might complicate the analysis of health effects experienced by SHAD veterans, especially if there were marked differences between the SHAD participants and the comparison group. Ideally, it would be possible to fully document the service histories of all members of the study population, but the necessary records are not available in electronic form. The best information available was from records of the Veterans Benefits Administration (VBA) of the Department of Veterans Affairs (VA). For veterans who apply for disability compensation,

**TABLE 4-1** Characteristics of Project SHAD Participants and the Comparison Population

| Characteristic | Project SHAD Participants N = 5,868 (%) | Comparison Population N = 6,753 (%) | Total N = 12,621 (%) |
|---|---|---|---|
| Year of Birth | | | |
| <1937 | 1,107 (18.8) | 1,193 (17.7) | 2,300 (18.2) |
| 1937-1946 | 3,514 (59.9) | 3,982 (59.0) | 7,496 (59.4) |
| >1946 | 925 (15.8) | 1,012 (15.0) | 1,937 (15.3) |
| Unknown | 322 (5.5) | 566 (8.4) | 888 (7.0) |
| Race[a] | | | |
| Nonwhite | 637 (13.1) | 491 (11.3) | 1,128 (12.2) |
| White | 4,241 (86.9) | 3,846 (88.7) | 8,087 (87.8) |
| Branch | | | |
| Navy | 5,066 (86.3) | 6,137 (90.9) | 11,203 (88.8) |
| Marines, other branches, and unknown | 802 (13.6) | 616 (9.1%) | 1,418 (11.2) |
| Rank | | | |
| Officer | 471 (8.0) | 496 (7.3) | 967 (7.7) |
| Enlisted | 5,394 (91.9) | 6,257 (92.7) | 11,651 (92.3) |
| Unknown | 3 | | 3 |
| Vietnam service among those filing for VA disability[b] | 1,018 (17.3) | 1,243 (18.4) | 2,261 (17.9) |
| Presumed or documented Agent Orange exposure among those filing for VA disability[c] | 475 (8.1) | 453 (6.7) | 928 (7.4) |

[a] Percentage is among those with known race. Race was unknown for 16.9 percent of SHAD participants and 35.8 percent of the comparison population.
[b] Vietnam service is defined as duty or visitation within the country of South Vietnam, including Navy veterans who entered inland waterways on ships, went ashore from offshore ships, or served only aboard offshore ships and never went ashore or entered inland waterways (Personal communication, J. Sampsel, Veterans Benefit Administration, March 12, 2014).
[c] Veterans with duty or visitation within the country of South Vietnam, including Navy veterans who entered inland waterways on ships or went ashore from offshore ships, qualify for a presumption of exposure to Agent Orange. A presumption of Agent Orange exposure also applies to veterans with service in certain military units on the Korean demilitarized zone during the Vietnam era. Veterans with service in other locations where testing and storage of Agent Orange occurred may also be designated as exposed if evidence shows that the veteran was directly involved (Personal communication, J. Sampsel, Veterans Benefit Administration, March 12, 2014).

VBA records include information on whether the veteran is considered to have service in Vietnam and whether the veteran is considered to have been exposed to Agent Orange, on the basis of documented exposure or presumed exposure because of the location of military service. The committee was reassured to find (see Table 4-1) that VBA records show similar percentages of the SHAD veterans and the comparison population with indicators for both Vietnam service and Agent Orange exposure.

## AVAILABILITY OF MORTALITY DATA

The analysis of the mortality experience of the study population considered both the timing of deaths and their underlying causes. The sources of mortality data for this study population are described in Chapter 3. As shown in Table 4-2, similar percentages of the SHAD test participants and comparison population were known to be dead or assumed to be alive as of December 31, 2011, which was the end of the follow-up period for this study. Roughly 68 percent of the SHAD participants and the comparison population were assumed alive at that time. Information on cause of death was available in each group for approximately 91 percent of those who had died.

## ALL-CAUSE MORTALITY

The mortality experience of the study population was assessed first for all deaths, regardless of the cause. A comparison of the timing of deaths among the SHAD participants and the comparison population was done using Kaplan-Meier survival analysis. This is a statistical technique that assesses the probability of surviving from one time interval to another. Because the various SHAD tests took place in different years the analysis is based on annual survival in the time since the first test in which a veteran was a participant. For the participants in the earliest tests (e.g., Eager Belle in early 1963), this period is approximately 48 years; for those who participated only in the final test (DTC 69-32 in spring 1969), the interval is approximately 42 years.

The committee found on the basis of the Kaplan-Meier analysis that the overall survival experience of the test participant and comparison populations was very similar (see Figure 4-1), and a statistical test (the log-rank test) showed that the small differences between the two curves were not statistically significant.

**TABLE 4-2** Vital Status and Availability of Data on Death for Project SHAD Participants and the Comparison Population as of December 31, 2011

| Vital Status and Death Data Available | Project SHAD Participants | Comparison Population | Total |
|---|---|---|---|
| Assumed alive | 3,975 (67.7%) | 4,574 (67.7%) | 8,549 (67.7%) |
| Known dead | 1,893 | 2,179 | 4,075 |
| *Date or fact of death only* | *162 (8.6%)* | *198 (9.1%)* | *360 (8.8%)* |
| *Cause of death available* | *1,731 (91.4%)* | *1,981 (90.9%)* | *3,712 (91.1%)* |
| Total population | 5,868 | 6,753 | 12,621 |

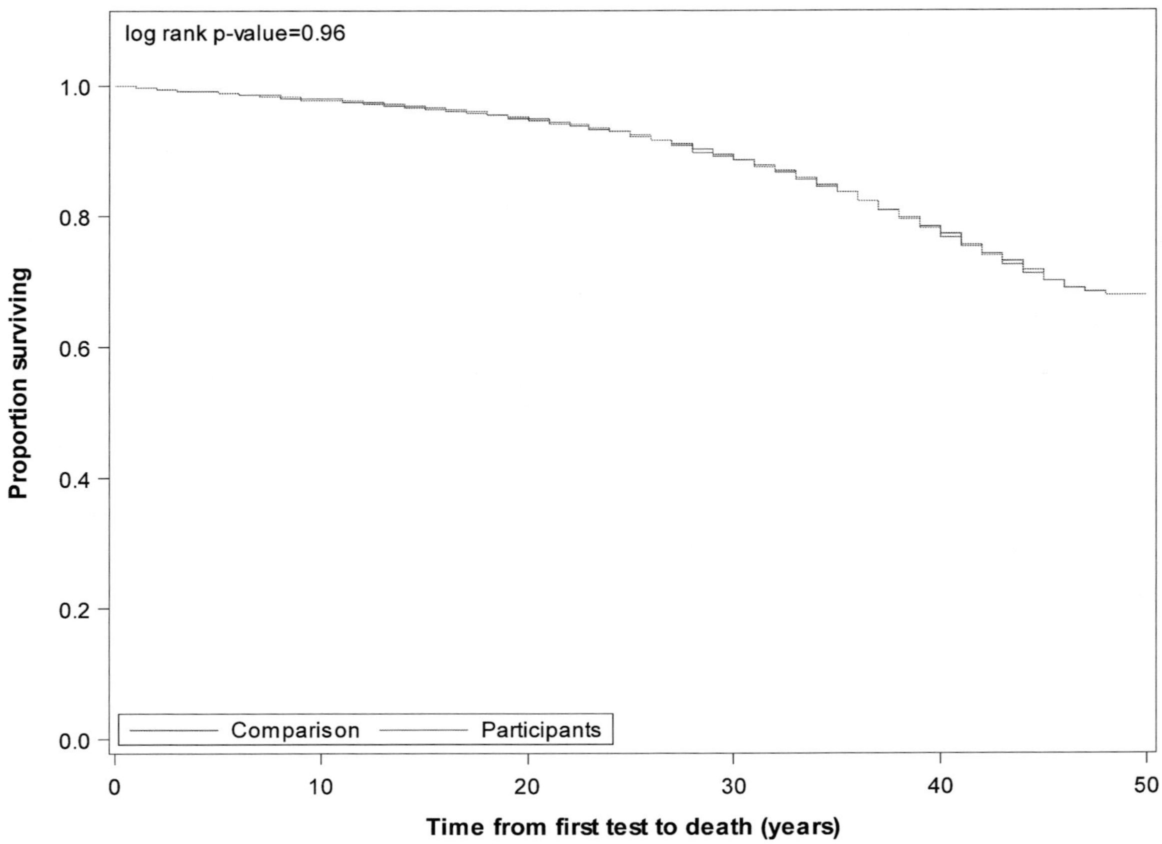


**FIGURE 4-1** Survival during the follow-up period by Project SHAD participant status. Statistical Analysis System (SAS) version 9.4 was used for the Kaplan-Meier analysis.

Another approach to comparing the overall mortality experience of the SHAD veterans with the comparison population makes use of the Cox proportional hazards model. This approach can also incorporate consideration of ("adjustment for") age at SHAD test, rank (officer versus enlisted), and service branch (Navy versus Marines and other) as well as SHAD participation. This analysis was used to assess all-cause mortality and (described below) cause-specific mortality. It was limited to subjects for whom the year of death was available. Use of the proportional hazards model assumes proportionality in the associated hazard functions (force of mortality). Proportionality was confirmed graphically by plotting the logarithm of cumulative hazard based on Kaplan-Meier estimates versus the logarithm of time. Detail about fitting the statistical model is provided in Appendix D.

As can be seen in Table 4-3, the SHAD participants and the comparison population did not differ significantly in overall mortality. This held true as well when the analysis was adjusted for age, rank, and service branch. Age, rank, and service branch each had a statistically significant association with total mortality. For example, enlisted personnel in the study population had a significantly higher risk of death than officers, whether or not they had been SHAD participants. Race is often included in analyses such as these. However, information on race was available for only 73 percent of the study population, with the percentage with

**TABLE 4-3** Survival Analysis Using Proportional Hazards Regression: All-Cause Mortality for the SHAD Participant and Comparison Populations

| Risk Factor | Unadjusted Hazard Ratio | 95% Confidence Interval | Adjusted Hazard Ratio[a] | 95% Confidence Interval |
|---|---|---|---|---|
| SHAD participation | | | | |
| Comparison population | 1 | | 1 | |
| Project SHAD participants | 1.01 | 0.88-1.16 | 0.94 | 0.85-1.04 |
| Age (years) | | | **1.09** | **1.09-1.10** |
| Rank | | | | |
| Officer | | | 1 | |
| Enlisted | | | **1.81** | **1.58-2.08** |
| Service branch | | | | |
| Navy | | | 1 | |
| Marines and other | | | **1.35** | **1.17-1.57** |

[a] All factors are adjusted simultaneously. For example, the adjusted hazard ratio for Project SHAD participants is adjusted for age, rank, and service branch. Ship ID was used in the model as a random effect to control for ship-clustering: estimated standard error for the random effects is 0.0059. SAS version 9.4 was used for all analyses.

unknown race greater among the comparison group (36 percent) than the SHAD test participants (17 percent), providing a compelling reason to exclude race in the analysis. The committee did not wish to omit those with missing data and did not have a good means to impute race. The committee did not observe differential exposure by race, and had no reason to anticipate a differential effect of exposure based upon race.

## CAUSE-SPECIFIC MORTALITY

The committee also explored whether SHAD participants may have been at increased risk of death from particular causes. Two approaches were used to look at cause-specific mortality. One approach, which was also used in the SHAD I study (IOM, 2007), relied on broad categories of causes of death that are used in the 9th and 10th revisions of the *International Classification of Diseases* (ICD-9 and ICD-10) (WHO, 2015). The mortality analysis also examined the specific causes of death that were identified from the review of the literature on potential health effects associated with exposure to some of the substances used in the SHAD tests. The ICD codes that correspond to the categories of causes of death are provided in Appendix F.

### Broad Categories of Causes of Death

The survival experiences of the SHAD test participants and the members of the comparison population were very similar for all the causes of death considered. Table 4-4 presents both the crude (unadjusted) hazard ratios and the hazard ratios adjusted for age and rank for each of the broad cause-of-death categories using Cox proportional hazard regression. The Project SHAD test participant population and comparison population had similar cause-specific

**TABLE 4-4** Proportional Hazards Regression for Broad Categories of Cause of Death for SHAD Participant and Comparison Populations (Cause of death available: Participants = 1,731; Comparison = 1,981)

| | Number of Deaths | | | | Enlisted Only<br>Number of Deaths | | |
|---|---|---|---|---|---|---|---|
| Cause of Death | SHAD Participants | Comparison Population | Unadjusted HR (95% CI) | Adjusted HR[a] (95% CI) | SHAD Participants | Comparison Population | Adjusted HR (95% CI)[b] |
| Infectious disease | 44 | 44 | 1.14 (0.72-1.80) | 1.08 (0.70-1.66) | 39 | 41 | 1.07 (0.68-1.68) |
| Cancer | 550 | 663 | 0.96 (0.81-1.13) | 0.93 (0.83-1.04) | 520 | 618 | 0.96 (0.85-1.08) |
| Endocrine/metabolic disease | 58 | 66 | 1.03 (0.68-1.55) | 1.00 (0.70-1.43) | 54 | 61 | 1.03 (0.71-1.50) |
| Neurocognitive disease | 23 | 31 | 0.85 (0.48-1.53) | 0.80 (0.45-1.44) | 19 | 31 | 0.66 (0.35-1.27) |
| Heart disease | 577 | 602 | 1.12 (0.95-1.32) | 1.09 (0.91-1.29) | 540 | 569 | 1.10 (0.91-1.32) |
| *Ischemic heart disease* | *346* | *374* | *1.08 (0.90-1.30)* | *1.05 (0.89-1.25)* | *321* | *354* | *1.06 (0.89-1.27)* |
| *Other heart disease* | *231* | *228* | *1.16 (0.92-1.46)* | *1.11 (0.87-1.42)* | *219* | *215* | *1.13 (0.86-1.48)* |
| Respiratory disease | 141 | 152 | 1.09 (0.83-1.42) | 1.04 (0.80-1.34) | 131 | 137 | 1.10 (0.85-1.43) |
| Digestive disease | 72 | 93 | 0.89 (0.62-1.28) | 0.87 (0.62-1.23) | 68 | 90 | 0.86 (0.61-1.22) |
| Injury/external causes | 141 | 193 | 0.85 (0.68-1.07) | 0.82 (0.65-1.03) | 132 | 189 | **0.78 (0.62-0.98)** |

NOTES: CI = confidence interval; HR = hazard ratio. See Appendix F for the ICD-9 codes that correspond to the categories of illness. SAS version 9.4 was used for all analyses.
[a] Adjusted for age, rank (officer/enlisted), and service branch.
[b] Adjusted for age only. Analysis takes into account competing risks.

mortality for most causes of death. The committee also evaluated enlisted and officer populations separately, aware of the possibility of differential exposures based upon experiences on the ships, as well as the socioeconomic differences that may accompany differences in rank. Examination of the enlisted and officer groups separately indicated statistically significantly fewer deaths from injury and external causes among the enlisted personnel in the SHAD participant population compared to the enlisted personnel in the comparison group. The committee did not pursue this result further because its interest was in the potential for increased rather than decreased risk among Project SHAD exposure groups.[1] No statistically significant differences were seen among the much smaller group of officers in this or any of the other analyses discussed in this chapter (data not shown).

[1] The reported statistical significance is the result of an implicit two-sided alternative of any difference between the SHAD population and the comparison population; it would not be observed if a one-sided alterantive of higher risk among SHAD population were explicitly used.

### Testing Hypotheses Regarding Specific Exposures

As described in Chapter 3, the committee's review of literature on the agents, simulants, tracers, and decontaminants used in the SHAD tests led to the formulation of hypotheses regarding the potential for increased risk of certain adverse health outcomes among SHAD veterans exposed to any of six substances: *Coxiella burnetii*, betapropriolactone, staphylococcal enterotoxin type B (SEB), *Escherichia coli*, sarin, and zinc cadmium sulfide. Because the individuals who served on the vessels involved in testing SEB were not identified, the committee could not test the hypotheses generated for this agent.

The vital status of Project SHAD veterans who participated in tests that used the remaining five substances is shown in Table 4-5. Comparison groups for these SHAD participants were identified as described in Chapter 3 and had served on similar ships deployed at the same time from a similar home port. Approximately 60 to 68 percent of the individuals in these exposure groups were assumed alive (not known to be dead) as of December 31, 2011.

**TABLE 4-5** Vital Status of SHAD Participants by Potential Exposure to Agents, Simulants, and Decontaminants for Which Health Outcomes Were Hypothesized

| Exposure and Vital Status | Project SHAD Participants | Comparison Group |
|---|---|---|
| *Coxiella burnetii* | | |
| Total group | 141 | 212 |
| Assumed alive | 84 (59.6%) | 138 (65.1%) |
| Total known dead | 57 (40.4%) | 74 (34.9%) |
| Cause of death available | 53 (37.6%) | 69 (32.5%) |
| Only date or fact of death available | 4 (2.8%) | 5 (2.4%) |
| Betapropiolactone | | |
| Total group | 595 | 607 |
| Assumed alive | 399 (67.1%) | 385 (63.4%) |
| Total known dead | 196 (32.9%) | 222 (36.6%) |
| Cause of death available | 178 (29.9%) | 195 (32.1%) |
| Only date or fact of death available | 18 (3.0%) | 27 (4.4%) |
| *Escherichia coli* | | |
| Total group | 141 | 228 |
| Assumed alive | 96 (68.1%) | 155 (68.0%) |
| Total known dead | 45 (31.9%) | 73 (32.0%) |
| Cause of death available | 43 (30.5%) | 68 (29.8%) |
| Only date or fact of death available | 2 (1.4%) | 5 (2.2%) |
| Sarin | | |
| Total group | 129 | 197 |
| Assumed alive | 80 (62.0%) | 127 (64.5%) |
| Total known dead | 49 (38.0%) | 70 (35.5%) |
| Cause of death available | 44 (34.1%) | 63 (32.0%) |
| Only date or fact of death available | 5 (3.9%) | 7 (3.6%) |
| Zinc cadmium sulfide | | |
| Total group | 681 | 773 |
| Assumed alive | 448 (65.8%) | 507 (65.6%) |
| Total known dead | 233 (34.2%) | 266 (34.4%) |
| Cause of death available | 214 (31.4%) | 242 (31.3%) |
| Only date or fact of death available | 19 (2.8%) | 24 (3.1%) |

## All-Cause Mortality for Selected Exposures

Before considering the specific health outcomes that the literature review suggested might be associated with the exposure experience of certain SHAD participants, the committee examined the overall survival patterns of the groups with those exposures. The analysis showed that these SHAD participants and their comparison groups were similar, with no statistically significant differences in survival for any of these exposure groups (see Table 4-6). Similarly, when the enlisted and officer groups were compared separately, the results were not statistically significant (officer data not shown).

**TABLE 4-6** Proportional Hazards Regression for All-Cause Mortality for SHAD Participants with Exposure to Selected Substances and the Comparison Groups

| Exposure and Risk Factor | Unadjusted Hazard Ratio (95% CI) | Adjusted Hazard Ratio[a] (95% CI) |
|---|---|---|
| *Coxiella burnetii* | | |
| Participant (n = 141, known dead = 57) versus comparison (n = 212, known dead = 74) | 1.37 (0.53-3.52) | 0.81 (0.24-2.69) |
| Enlisted (P, n = 122, known dead = 50 versus Enlisted (C, n = 192, known dead = 71) | 1.26 (0.45-3.49) | 0.74 (0.19-2.83) |
| Betapropiolactone | | |
| Participant (n = 595, known dead = 196) versus comparison (n = 607, known dead = 222) | 0.94 (0.73-1.22) | 0.97 (0.79-1.19) |
| Enlisted (P, n = 546, known dead = 183) versus Enlisted (C, n = 555, known dead = 210) | 0.92 (0.71-1.20) | 1.00 (0.77-1.30) |
| *Escherichia coli* | | |
| Participant (n = 141, known dead = 45) versus comparison (n = 228, known dead = 73) | 1.01 (0.69-1.48) | 0.94 (0.64-1.38) |
| Enlisted (P, n = 132, known dead = 40 versus Enlisted (C, n = 217, known dead = 70) | 0.94 (0.63-1.40) | 0.91 (0.61-1.36) |
| Sarin | | |
| Participant (n = 129, known dead = 49) versus comparison (n = 197, known dead = 70) | 1.11 (0.75-1.63) | 1.07 (0.73-1.57) |
| Enlisted (P, n = 114, known dead = 43) versus Enlisted (C, n = 176, known dead = 66) | 1.04 (0.70-1.56) | 1.04 (0.70-1.56) |
| Zinc cadmium sulfide | | |
| Participant (n = 681, known dead = 233) versus comparison (n = 773, known dead = 266) | 1.01 (0.84-1.22) | 0.93 (0.75-1.15) |
| Enlisted (P, n = 621, known dead = 215 versus Enlisted (C, n = 716, known dead = 252) | 1.03 (0.82-1.29) | 0.91 (0.66-1.25) |

NOTES: CI = confidence interval. Ship ID was used in the model as random effect. SAS version 9.4 was used for all analyses.

[a] Adjusted for age and rank (officer/enlisted). Enlisted and officer groups adjusted only for age.

## Mortality from Health Outcomes with a Hypothesized Association with Certain SHAD Test Exposures

For each of the six exposures for which the potential for certain adverse health outcomes was hypothesized, the number of deaths attributed to these conditions was tabulated (see Table 4-7). Kaplan-Meier analyses of the survival experience of exposed SHAD participants found no statistically significant difference from the experience of the comparison groups. Similarly, a proportional hazards analysis that included adjustment for age and rank found no statistically significant excess risk among SHAD participants (see Table 4-8) for the two categories for which there were sufficient number of cases to pursue the analysis (i.e., exposure to betapropriolactone or zinc cadmium sulfide). When examined separately, the findings were similar in the enlisted members of these exposure groups.

**TABLE 4-7** Mortality from Hypothesized Health Outcomes for SHAD Participants with Exposure to Specific Agents and the Comparison Groups

| Exposure and Hypothesized Health Outcome | Number of Deaths | |
|---|---|---|
| | SHAD Participants | Comparison Group |
| *Coxiella burnetii* (Total group) | (141) | (212) |
| Endocarditis | 0 | 0 |
| Fatigue | 0 | 0 |
| Chronic hepatitis | 0 | 0 |
| Osteomyelitis | 0 | 0 |
| Vascular infection | 0 | 0 |
| Betapropiolactone | (595) | (607) |
| All cancer | 51 | 61 |
| *Escherichia coli* | (141) | (228) |
| Irritable bowel syndrome | 0 | 0 |
| Sarin | (129) | (197) |
| Neurological effects: CNS | 0 | 0 |
| Neurological effects: PNS | 0 | 0 |
| Neurological effects: Hearing loss | 0 | 0 |
| Psychological symptoms | 0 | 0 |
| Zinc cadmium sulfide | (681) | (773) |
| Lung cancer | 33 | 28 |
| Chronic kidney disease: Broad definition | ≤10 | ≤10 |
| Chronic kidney disease: Narrow definition | ≤10 | ≤10 |

NOTES: CNS = central nervous system; PNS = peripheral nervous system. Cell sizes smaller than 11 were reported as "≤10" to prevent identification of any individual.

**TABLE 4-8** Survival Analysis Using Proportional Hazards Regression: Cause-Specific Mortality for Hypothesized Health Outcomes (Adjusted for Age and Rank)

| Potential Exposure/ Cause of Death | Number of Deaths | | Unadjusted HR (95% CI) | Adjusted HR[a] (95% CI) | Enlisted Only |
|---|---|---|---|---|---|
| | SHAD Participants | Comparison Group | | | Adjusted HR[b] (95% CI) |
| Betapropiolactone and cancer | 51 | 61 | 0.84 (0.58-1.22) | 0.86 (0.53-1.41) | 0.87 (0.54-1.41) |
| Zinc cadmium sulfide and lung cancer | 33 | 28 | 1.76 (0.68-4.55) | 1.44 (0.66-3.17) | 1.37 (0.60-3.10) |

NOTES: CI = confidence interval; HR = hazard ratio. SAS version 9.4 was used in all analyses.
[a] Adjusted for age and rank (officer/enlisted).
[b] Adjusted for age only.

## Examining an Association Between Number of Potential Exposures and Mortality from Specified Health Outcomes

The committee also examined the possibility that the numbers of times SHAD test participants were potentially exposed to the substances of interest was associated with an increase in risk of mortality. The committee grouped the test participants into groups depending upon the distribution of the numbers of test trials that individuals were exposed to. Details of the basis for this grouping are provided in Appendix D. Table 4-9 shows the hazard ratios and confidence intervals for risk of mortality from any cause by numbers of exposures to the substances. The comparison is with people on similar ships without any SHAD test exposures. The numbers of exposures to *C. burnetii* and sarin were too similar across the exposed groups to justify establishing higher and lower levels of exposure.

## Exploratory Analyses of Mortality

In addition to testing the hypotheses regarding specific health outcomes that were identified as potentially associated with exposure to certain substances used in Project SHAD, the committee examined mortality for broader exposure groupings and other subgroups of special interest. These groupings were defined as (1) exposure to any biological test substance; (2) exposure to any chemical test substance (except trioctyl phosphate [TOF]); (3) exposure to any decontaminant; (4) exposure to TOF, which was used only in Test 69-10; (5) service on the light tugs or as Project SHAD staff on the USS *Granville S. Hall*, and (6) service on the USS *George Eastman*. These groups are not necessarily mutually exclusive. Because many SHAD tests included the use of multiple substances (e.g., a biological agent such as *B. globigii* and a chemical tracer such as zinc cadmium sulfide), a given SHAD veteran may be included in more than one of these groups. However, the men who were exposed to TOF in Test 69-10 had no other reported exposures.

The committee also reviewed the mortality of crews of each of the individual vessels and other units involved in Project SHAD to see if any unit warranted additional scrutiny. This crude analysis suggested no atypical mortality for any specific unit that would warrant additional follow up (data not shown).

**TABLE 4-9** Proportional Hazards Regression for Overall Mortality for Groups with Lower and Higher Exposure to Selected Substances and the Comparison Groups

| Exposure and Exposure Frequency | Assumed Alive | Deceased | Unadjusted Hazard Ratio (95% CI) | Adjusted Hazard Ratio[a] (95% CI) |
|---|---|---|---|---|
| Betapropiolactone | | | | |
| 0 exposures (comparison group) | 385 | 222 | 1 | 1 |
| 1 to 5 | 156 | 66 | 0.89 (0.61-1.31) | 0.94 (0.68-1.30) |
| ≥6 | 243 | 130 | 0.99 (0.72-1.37) | 1.02 (0.78-1.33) |
| Standard error of Ship ID (used as a random effect) | | | (0.0262) | (0.0187) |
| Zinc cadmium sulfide | | | | |
| 0 exposures | 507 | 266 | 1 | 1 |
| 1 to 29 | 268 | 132 | 0.95 (0.76-1.18) | 0.98 (0.70-1.38) |
| ≥30 | 180 | 101 | 1.11 (0.87-1.40) | 0.88 (0.64-1.22) |
| Standard error of Ship ID (used as a random effect) | | | (0.0141) | (0.0261) |

NOTES: CI = confidence interval. Ship ID was used in the model as random effect. SAS version 9.4 was used in all analyses.
[a] Adjusted for age and rank (officer/enlisted).

Information on the vital status of the members of these exposure groups is presented in Table 4-10. Except for the TOF group, and those who served on the tugs and Project SHAD technical staff, roughly two-thirds of both the SHAD participants and the comparison groups are assumed to be alive as of December 31, 2011. Approximately three-fourths of the TOF group were assumed to be alive. This group participated in Test 69-10, which was one of the last two SHAD tests, and the participants and comparison group are younger on average than the other groups. Across all exposure groups, there were 3-4 percent of subjects for whom only a date of death or fact of death was available, with the exception of the tugs where this was close to 5 percent.

### All-Cause Mortality for Subgroups of Special Interest

The committee examined all-cause mortality among the SHAD veterans in the subgroups of special interest and their respective comparison groups. As shown in Table 4-11, mortality among the members of the special subgroups was not significantly different from their comparison groups. Similarly, stratifying the groups on the basis of rank (officer and enlisted) resulted in no statistically significant differences. Members of the tug and Project SHAD technical staff groups had higher crude mortality when compared to the other members of the crew of the USS *Granville S. Hall* (internal control) and to the crew of the comparison vessel for the USS *Granville S. Hall* (external control), but this was accounted for by a difference in age in the two groups (data not shown) and the difference was not statistically significant after adjustment for age.

**TABLE 4-10** Vital Status and Availability of Data on Death for Subgroups of Special Interest and Their Comparison Groups as of December 31, 2011

| Exposure Group and Vital Status | Project SHAD Participants | Comparison Group | |
|---|---|---|---|
| **Any Biological Substance** | | | |
| Total group | 3,050 | 3,530 | |
| Assumed alive | 2,003 (65.7%) | 2,311 (65.5%) | |
| Total known dead | 1,047 (34.3%) | 1,219 (34.5%) | |
| Cause of death available | 965 (31.6%) | 1,113 (31.5%) | |
| Only date or fact of death available | 82 (2.7%) | 106 (3.0%) | |
| **Any Chemical Substance (except Trioctyle Phosphate)** | | | |
| Total group | 2,536 | 2,804 | |
| Assumed alive | 1,694 (66.70%) | 1,916 (68.3%) | |
| Total known dead | 842 (33.2%) | 888 (31.7%) | |
| Cause of death available | 775 (30.6%) | 818 (29.2%) | |
| Only date or fact of death available | 67 (2.6%) | 70 (2.5%) | |
| **Any Decontaminant** | | | |
| Total group | 730 | 782 | |
| Assumed alive | 493 (67.5%) | 517 (66.1%) | |
| Total known dead | 237 (32.5%) | 265 (33.1%) | |
| Cause of death available | 217 (29.7%) | 235 (30.1%) | |
| Only date or fact of death available | 20 (2.7%) | 30 (3.8%) | |
| **Trioctyl Phosphate** | | | |
| Total group | 861 | 869 | |
| Assumed alive | 656 (76.2%) | 668 (76.9%) | |
| Total known dead | 205 (23.8%) | 201 (23.1%) | |
| Cause of death available | 182 (21.1%) | 172 (19.8%) | |
| Only date or fact of death available | 23 (2.8%) | 29 (3.3%) | |
| **Tugs and Project SHAD Technical Staff** | | **Internal Comparison** | **External Comparison** |
| Total group | 103 | 127 | 210 |
| Assumed alive | 59 (57.2%) | 86 (67.7%) | 136 (64.8) |
| Total known dead | 44 (42.7%) | 41 (32.3%) | 74 (35.2) |
| Cause of death available | 39 (37.8%) | 38 (29.9%) | 69 (32.9) |
| Only date or fact of death available | 5 (4.9%) | 3 (2.4%) | 5 (2.4) |
| **Crew of the USS *George Eastman*** | | | |
| Total group | 356 | 47 | |
| Assumed alive | 228 (64.0%) | 506 (69.1%) | |
| Total known dead | 128 (36.0%) | 241 (32.3%) | |
| Cause of death available | 119 (33.4%) | 218 (29.2%) | |
| Only date or fact of death available | 9 (2.5%) | 23 (3.1%) | |

**TABLE 4-11** Survival Analysis Using Proportional Hazards Regression: All-Cause Mortality for SHAD Participants Versus Comparison Groups

| Exposure Group and Risk Factor | Unadjusted Hazard Ratio (95% CI) | Adjusted Hazard Ratio (95% CI) |
|---|---|---|
| Any Biological Test Substance | | |
| Participant (n = 3,050, known dead = 1,047) versus comparison (n = 3,530, known dead = 1,219 with known date of death) | 1.02 (0.88-1.20) | 0.96[a] (0.86-1.08) |
| Enlisted (P, n = 2,793, known dead = 981) versus Enlisted (C, n = 3,257, known dead = 1,158) | 1.01 (0.88-1.17) | 0.97[b] (0.87-1.09) |
| Any Chemical Test Substance (excluding TOF) | | |
| Participant (n = 2,536, known dead = 842) versus comparison (n = 2,804, known dead = 888) | 1.11 (0.94-1.31) | 1.03[a] (0.91-1.17) |
| Enlisted (P, n = 2,319, known dead = 786) versus Enlisted (C, n = 2,596, known dead = 844) | 1.10 (0.95-1.28) | 1.04[b] (0.91-1.18) |
| Any Decontaminant | | |
| Participant (n = 730, known dead = 237) versus comparison (n = 782, known dead = 265) | 1.01 (0.79-1.29) | 1.08[a] (0.83-1.41) |
| Enlisted (P, n = 668, known dead = 220) versus Enlisted (C, n = 709, known dead = 252) | 0.97 (0.77-1.21) | 1.07[b] (0.81-1.42) |
| Trioctyl Phosphate | | |
| Participant (n = 861, known dead = 205) versus comparison (n = 869, known dead = 201) | 1.08 (0.83-1.39) | 0.90[a] (0.60-1.35) |
| Enlisted (P, n = 822, known dead = 199) versus Enlisted (C, n = 827, known dead = 196) | 1.06 (0.83-1.37) | 0.90[b] (0.61-1.33) |
| Tugs or Project SHAD Technical Staff | | |
| Participant (n = 103, known dead = 44) versus **internal** comparison (n = 127, known dead = 41)[c] | **1.83 (1.08-3.09)** | 1.12[a] (0.65-1.93) |
| Participant (n = 103, known dead = 44) versus **external** comparison (n = 210, known dead = 74)[d] | 1.20 (0.40-3.60) | 0.78[a] (0.22-2.78) |
| Enlisted (P, n = 88, known dead = 39) versus **internal** comparison Enlisted (C, n = 115, known dead = 38)[c] | **1.97 (1.13-3.45)** | 1.20[b] (0.67-2.14) |
| Enlisted (P, n = 88, known dead = 39) versus **external** comparison Enlisted (C, n = 191, known dead = 71)[d] | 1.19 (0.37-3.87) | 0.73[b] (0.20-2.70) |
| Crew of the USS *George Eastman* | | |
| Participant (n = 356, known dead = 128) versus comparison (n = 747, known dead = 241) | 1.18 (0.92-1.52) | 1.19[a] (0.95-1.49) |
| Enlisted (P, n = 314, known dead = 117) versus Enlisted (C, n = 697, known dead = 231) | 1.21 (0.87-1.69) | 1.18[b] (0.94-1.49) |

NOTES: CI = confidence interval. SAS version 9.4 was used in all analyses.
[a] Adjusted for age and officer/enlisted.
[b] Adjusted for age only. Ship ID is used as random term.
[c] Comparison is an "internal control" made up of the crew of the USS *Granville S. Hall* who were not part of the Project SHAD technical staff.
[d] Comparison is an "external control" made up of the crew of the USS *Interceptor*, which was the comparison ship for the USS *Granville S. Hall*.

## Examining an Association Between Number of Potential Exposures and Mortality in Subgroups of Special Interest

The committee also examined the possibility that the numbers of times SHAD test participants were potentially exposed to the substances of interest was associated with an increase in risk of mortality. The committee grouped the test participants into two or three groups, depending upon the distribution of the numbers of test trials that individuals were exposed to. Details of the basis for this grouping are provided in Appendix D. Table 4-12 shows the hazard ratios and confidence intervals for risk of mortality from any cause associated with varying numbers of potential exposures to the substances listed for each the special subgroups considered, compared with people on similar ships without any SHAD exposures. Such groupings were not feasible for groups exposed to TOF and for the other special subgroups listed in Table 4-10 because the people involved were present for similar numbers of potential exposures.

**TABLE 4-12** Hazard Ratios for Overall Mortality for Groups in the Subgroups of Special Interest with Lower and Higher Potential Exposure

| Potential Exposure and Number of Exposures | Assumed Alive | Deceased | Unadjusted Hazard Ratio (95% CI) | Adjusted Hazard Ratio[a] (95% CI) |
|---|---|---|---|---|
| Any Biological Test Substance | | | | |
| 0 (comparison group) | 2,311 | 1,219 | 1 | 1 |
| 1 to 53 | 1,823 | 946 | 1.02 (0.87-1.20) | 0.98 (0.86-1.11) |
| ≥54 | 180 | 101 | 1.03 (0.80-1.33) | 0.89 (0.70-1.14) |
| Standard error of ship ID (used as a random effect) | | | | (0.0065) |
| Any Chemical Test Substance (excluding TOF) | | | | |
| 0 | 1,916 | 888 | 1 | 1 |
| 1 to 20 | 1,216 | 596 | 1.05 (0.88-1.26) | 1.05 (0.91-1.21) |
| ≥21 | 478 | 246 | 1.25 (1.00-1.55) | 0.99 (0.82-1.19) |
| Standard error of ship ID (used as a random effect) | | | | (0.0076) |
| Any Decontaminant | | | | |
| 0 | 517 | 265 | 1 | 1 |
| 1 to 5 | 162 | 82 | 1.05 (0.76-1.46) | 1.07 (0.76-1.52) |
| 6 to 10 | 250 | 132 | 1.08 (0.80-1.48) | 1.15 (0.83-1.59) |
| ≥11 | 81 | 23 | 0.70 (0.42-1.14) | 0.88 (0.53-1.47) |
| Standard error of ship ID (used as a random effect) | | | | (0.0256) |

NOTES: CI = confidence interval; TOF = trioctyl phosphate. SAS version 9.4 was used in all analyses.
[a] All factors are adjusted simulatenously for age and rank. Ship ID is used as random term.

### Cause-Specific Mortality for Subgroups of Special Interest

Analysis of cause-specific mortality for the group of participants exposed to any biological test substances (listed in Box 3-1) indicated a decreased risk of death from injury and external causes for all of the participants when analyzed as a group, and for enlisted participants but not officers when assessed separately (see Table 4-13). The committee did not pursue this result further because its interest was in the potential for increased rather than decreased risk among Project SHAD exposure groups.[2] After adjustment for age and rank, no statistically significant differences were found for those exposed to any chemical test substance (except TOF), any decontaminant, or TOF (also adjusted for service branch). Nor were there significant differences for the men who served on the tugs or were part of the Project SHAD technical staff. There was a statistically significant increase in the hazard ratio for heart disease mortality for the crew of the USS *George Eastman*. However, when the committee applied an adjustment to take into account the multiple tests it carried out to compare the mortality of the USS *George Eastman* crew with the comparison group (tests to compare mortality from cancer, heart disease, and respiratory disease), the result no longer attained statistical significance. Additional details of this adjustment are provided in Appendix D.

**TABLE 4-13** Survival Analysis Using Proportional Hazards Regression: Cause-Specific Mortality for SHAD Participant Subgroups of Special Interest Versus Comparison Groups

| Exposure Group and Cause of Death | Deaths: SHAD Participants | Deaths: Comparison Group | Unadjusted HR (95% CI) | Adjusted HR[a] (95% CI) | Enlisted Only Adjusted HR[b] (95% CI) |
|---|---|---|---|---|---|
| Any Biological Test Substance (SHAD participants n = 3,050, comparison n = 3,530) | | | | | |
| Cancer | 326 | 393 | 0.98 (0.80-1.20) | 0.91 (0.79-1.06) | 0.94 (0.81-1.10) |
| Heart disease | 312 | 336 | 1.06 (0.85-1.32) | 1.03 (0.83-1.27) | 1.03 (0.81-1.31) |
| *Ischemic heart disease* | *193* | *219* | *1.02 (0.81-1.29)* | *0.99 (0.77-1.27)* | *0.98 (0.75-1.27)* |
| *Other heart disease* | *119* | *117* | *1.12 (0.80-1.57)* | *1.11 (0.82-1.51)* | *1.16 (0.82-1.64)* |
| Respiratory disease | 78 | 93 | 0.96 (0.68-1.34) | 0.95 (0.65-1.39) | 1.00 (0.67-1.47) |
| Endocrine and metabolic disease | 33 | 33 | 1.15 (0.71-1.87) | 1.17 (0.72-1.91) | 1.11 (0.68-1.83) |
| Injury/external causes | 69 | 106 | 0.75 (0.55-1.02) | **0.72 (0.53-0.97)** | **0.69 (0.50-0.94)** |
| Infectious disease | 26 | 20 | 1.49 (0.75-2.98) | 1.32 (0.68-2.53) | 1.34 (0.66-2.70) |
| Neurocognitive disease | 14 | 16 | 0.99 (0.43-2.26) | 0.92 (0.41-2.08) | 0.67 (0.25-1.79) |
| Digestive disease | 38 | 43 | 1.03 (0.62-1.71) | 0.99 (0.62-1.58) | 0.98 (0.61-1.56) |
| Any Chemical Test Substance (excluding TOF) (SHAD participants n = 2,536, comparison n = 2,804) | | | | | |
| Cancer | 244 | 256 | 1.10 (0.89-1.35) | 1.02 (0.86-1.22) | 1.06 (0.88-1.28) |
| Heart disease | 257 | 264 | 1.10 (0.89-1.35) | 1.05 (0.89-1.25) | 1.07 (0.90-1.28) |
| *Ischemic heart disease* | *158* | *170* | *1.06 (0.83-1.35)* | *1.01 (0.81-1.25)* | *1.02 (0.81-1.27)* |

[2] The reported statistical significance is the result of an implicit two-sided alternative of any difference between the SHAD population and the comparison population: it would not be observed if a one-sided alterantive of higher risk among SHAD population were explicitly used.

| Exposure Group and Cause of Death | Deaths: SHAD Participants | Deaths: Comparison Group | Unadjusted HR (95% CI) | Adjusted HR[a] (95% CI) | Enlisted Only Adjusted HR[b] (95% CI) |
|---|---|---|---|---|---|
| *Other heart disease* | *99* | *94* | *1.15 (0.81-1.64)* | *1.13 (0.83-1.53* | *1.16 (0.86-1.58)* |
| Respiratory disease | 65 | 57 | 1.28 (0.85-1.93) | 1.21 (0.82-1.77) | 1.24 (0.84-1.85) |
| Endocrine and metabolic disease | 26 | 32 | 0.92 (0.55-1.54) | 0.88 (0.52-1.48) | 0.85 (0.50-1.47) |
| Injury/external causes | 70 | 78 | 1.01 (0.74-1.44) | 1.01 (0.71-1.44) | 0.93 (0.67-1.31) |
| Infectious disease | 18 | 15 | 1.35 (0.68-2.69) | 1.09 (0.53-2.22) | 1.04 (0.49-2.21) |
| Neurocognitive disease | ≤10 | 15 | 0.53 (0.22-1.29) | 0.51 (0.21-1.25) | 0.44 (0.17-1.15) |
| Digestive disease | 34 | 37 | 1.04 (0.64-1.70) | 0.98 (0.61-1.57) | 0.93 (0.57-1.51) |
| Any Decontaminant (SHAD participants n = 730, comparison n = 782) | | | | | |
| Cancer | 65 | 76 | 0.91 (0.64-1.29) | 0.93 (0.60-1.44) | 0.92 (0.56-1.49) |
| Heart disease | 74 | 75 | 1.10 (0.66-1.83) | 1.22(0.76-1.96) | 1.24 (0.73-2.11) |
| *Ischemic heart disease* | *52* | *47* | *1.21 (0.71-2.04)* | *1.35 (0.84-2.18)* | *1.33 (0.81-2.20)* |
| *Other heart disease* | *22* | *28* | *0.91 (0.38-2.22)* | *0.99 (0.39-2.46)* | *1.02 (0.41-2.56)* |
| Respiratory disease | 21 | 22 | 1.09 (0.45-2.64 | 1.17 (0.49-2.77) | 1.16 (0.50-2.71) |
| Endocrine and metabolic disease | ≤10 | ≤10 | 1.43 (0.49-4.11) | 1.56 (0.54-4.51) | 1.41 (0.47-4.22) |
| Injury/external causes | 14 | 20 | 0.76 (0.35-1.64) | 0.76 (0.35-1.66) | 0.82 (0.36-1.86) |
| Infectious disease | ≤10 | ≤10 | 1.65 (0.43-6.39) | 1.63 (0.41-6.40) | 1.49 (0.24-9.18) |
| Neurocognitive disease | ≤10 | ≤10 | 0.53 (0.10-2.91) | 0.67 (0.12-3.68) | 0.67 (0.12-3.68) |
| Digestive disease | 11 | ≤10 | 1.92 (0.49-7.59) | 1.89 (0.50-7.22) | 1.63 (0.40-6.60) |
| Trioctyl Phosphate (SHAD participants n = 861, comparison n = 869) | | | | | |
| Cancer | 49 | 59 | 0.83 0.54-1.30 | 0.73 (0.40-1.35) | 0.72 (0.39-1.31) |
| Heart disease | 74 | 49 | 1.46 0.83-2.57 | 1.22 (0.64-2.33) | 1.19 (0.64-2.23) |
| *Ischemic heart disease* | *44* | *26* | ***1.71 (1.03-2.84)*** | *1.47 (0.73-2.96)* | *1.45 (0.77-2.77)* |
| *Other heart disease* | *30* | *23* | *1.29 (0.67-2.49)* | *1.07 (0.53-2.18)* | *1.03 (0.48-2.23)* |
| Respiratory disease | 14 | ≤10 | 2.37 (0.91-6.16) | 1.68 (0.64-4.44) | 2.52 (0.82-7.72) |
| Endocrine and metabolic disease | ≤10 | ≤10 | 2.02 (0.51-8.08) | 2.39 (0.48-11.86) | 2.39 (0.48-11.86) |
| Injury/external causes | 15 | 18 | 0.94 (0.35-2.51) | 0.81 (0.31-2.07) | 0.81 (0.31-2.07) |
| Infectious disease | ≤10 | ≤10 | 0.45 (0.12-1.73) | 0.47 (0.14-1.63) | 0.47 (0.14-1.63) |
| Neurocognitive disease | ≤10 | ≤10 | 0.67 (0.11-4.01) | 0.53 (0.09-3.15) | 0.53 (0.09-3.15) |
| Digestive disease | ≤10 | 14 | 0.45 (0.13-1.58) | 0.34 (0.10-1.12) | 0.34 (0.10-1.12) |
| Tugs and Project SHAD Technical Staff (n = 103) | | | | | |
| *Comparison to Internal Controls*[c] (n = 127) | | | | | |
| Cancer | 22 | 19 | 2.00 (0.99-4.04) | 1.27 (0.61-2.66) | 1.33 (0.60-2.94) |
| Heart disease | ≤10 | ≤10 | 1.85 (0.67-5.14) | 1.08 (0.38-3.08) | 0.90 (0.31-2.62) |
| *Ischemic heart disease* | *≤10* | *≤10* | ***4.18 (1.16-15.01)*** | *2.56 (0.69-9.56)* | *2.20 (0.57-8.49)* |
| *Other heart disease* | *≤10* | *≤10* | *0.16 (0.01-3.44)* | *0.11 (0.01-1.83)* | *0.11 (0.01-1.83)* |

| Exposure Group and Cause of Death | Deaths: SHAD Participants | Deaths: Comparison Group | Unadjusted HR (95% CI) | Adjusted HR[a] (95% CI) | Enlisted Only Adjusted HR[b] (95% CI) |
|---|---|---|---|---|---|
| Respiratory disease | ≤10 | ≤10 | 1.96 (0.33-11.76) | 0.92 (0.15-5.67) | 2.09 (0.21-20.35) |
| *Comparison to External Controls*[d] (n = 210) | | | | | |
| Cancer | 22 | 18 | 2.54 (0.77-8.38) | 1.86 (048-7.20) | 1.63 (0.34-7.82) |
| Heart disease | ≤10 | 26 | 0.71 (0.17-2.90) | 0.47 (0.11-1.92) | 0.43 (0.13-1.46) |
| *Ischemic heart disease* | *≤10* | *18* | *0.80 (0.14-4.60)* | *0.52 (0.08-3.28)* | *0.49 (0.09-2.60)* |
| *Other heart disease* | *≤10* | *≤100* | *0.34 (0.01-13.33)* | *0.21 (0.01-5.91)* | *0.21 (0.01-5.91)* |
| Respiratory disease | ≤10 | ≤10 | 0.78 (0.21-2.88) | 0.42 (0.11-1.61) | 0.42 (0.11-1.61) |
| USS *George Eastman* (SHAD participants n = 356,comparison n = 747) | | | | | |
| Cancer | 26 | 65 | 0.87 (0.55-1.37) | 0.84 (0.53-1.34) | 0.89 (0.55-1.44) |
| Heart disease | 49 | 72 | 1.47 (0.98-2.21) | **1.48 (1.03-2.14)**[e] | **1.46 (1.01-2.12)**[e] |
| *Ischemic heart disease* | *34* | *47* | *1.56 (1.00-2.43)* | *1.55 (0.99-2.42)* | *1.52 (0.97-2.40)* |
| *Other heart disease* | *15* | *25* | *1.29 (0.64-2.64)* | *1.35 (0.71-2.57)* | *1.35 (0.71-2.56)* |
| Respiratory disease | ≤10 | 24 | 0.82 (0.31-2.15) | 0.79 (0.37-1.70) | 0.68 (0.29-1.58) |

NOTES: CI = confidence interval; TOF = trioctyl phosphate. Cell sizes smaller than 11 were reported as ≤10 to prevent identification of any individual. SAS version 9.4 was used in all analyses.

[a] Adjusted for age and officer/enlisted. Ship ID used as a random term. Analyses of the group exposed to TOF were also adjusted for service branch (Navy versus Marines and other).

[b] Adjusted for age only. Ship ID is used as random term.

[c] Comparison is an "internal control" made up of the crew of the USS *Granville S. Hall* who were not part of the Project SHAD technical staff.

[d] Comparison is an "external control" made up of the crew of the USS *Interceptor*, which was the comparison ship for the USS *Granville S. Hall.*

[e] P-values under the alternative of an odds ratio greater than 1 were adjusted for an overall false discovery rate (FDR) of 5 percent, taking into account three tests; after this adjustment the increase in heart disease risk was no longer statistically significant at the 5 percent FDR level.

## REFERENCES

IOM (Institute of Medicine). 2007. *Long-term health effects of participation in Project SHAD (Shipboard Hazard and Defense).* Washington, DC: The National Academies Press.

WHO (World Health Organization). 2015. *International Classification of Diseases (ICD).* http://www.who.int/classifications/icd/en/ (accessed August 4, 2015).

# 5

# Morbidity Results

The committee used information on diagnoses received by Shipboard Hazard and Defense (SHAD) test veterans and the comparison population to assess whether morbidity differed in the two groups. These data came from diagnoses recorded in Medicare (Parts A and B) claims for inpatient and outpatient care provided on a fee-for-service basis and from diagnoses recorded in Veterans Health Administration (VHA) records for inpatient and outpatient care, as described in Chapter 3. The committee carried out analyses of the overall population and tested specific hypotheses suggested by literature reviews on the agents, tracers, simulants, and decontaminants used in the SHAD tests.

## DATA FROM MEDICARE AND THE VETERANS HEALTH ADMINISTRATION

An important source of information on illness in the study population was in records of claims made for inpatient or outpatient care through the Medicare system. People become eligible for Medicare insurance in the year in which they turn 65, or when designated as eligible for disability through the Social Security Administration. These records provide information about days of hospitalization and diagnoses reported as part of the claim for the health services provided. Table 5-1 shows percentages of the Project SHAD participant and comparison populations enrolled in the fee-for-service form of Medicare Part A or B during 1999-2011, the period for which data were obtained. Approximately similar proportions of both groups were enrolled, starting at about 9 percent in 1999 and increasing to nearly 40 percent by 2011. However, an evaluation using logistic regression found the enrollment levels of Project SHAD participants were statistically significantly higher than those in the comparison group over the period of 13 years, and the SHAD participants also had statistically significantly higher annual increases in enrollment than the comparison group.

The other source of morbidity data was records of health care encounters with VHA. In contrast to Medicare, which has an identifiable "enrolled" population, eligibility for VHA services can vary depending on the nature of the veteran's military service, medical condition, and income status. Therefore the committee considered a record of any diagnosis in inpatient or outpatient records to be an indication that the individual was a user of the Department of Veterans Affairs (VA) health care services. Table 5-2 provides counts and percentages of Project

**TABLE 5-1** Enrollment in Medicare Fee-for-Service Among Project SHAD Participant and Comparison Populations, 1999-2011

| | Enrolled in Fee-for-Service Medicare (%) | | |
|---|---|---|---|
| Year | Project SHAD Participants N = 5,868 | Comparison Population N = 6,753 | |
| 1999 | 538 (9.2) | 623 (9.2) | Test for differential Medicare enrollment between SHAD participants and comparison group was based on a logistic regression with over-dispersion[a]; (one-sided) p-value = 0.0005 for additional annual increases in enrollment among SHAD participants. |
| 2000 | 606 (10.3) | 652 (9.7) | |
| 2001 | 709 (12.1) | 789 (11.7) | |
| 2002 | 853 (14.5) | 995 (14.7) | |
| 2003 | 980 (16.7) | 1,114 (16.5) | |
| 2004 | 1,100 (18.7) | 1,252 (18.5) | |
| 2005 | 1,223 (20.8) | 1,380 (20.4) | |
| 2006 | 1,396 (23.8) | 1,551 (23.0) | |
| 2007 | 1,611 (27.5) | 1,783 (26.4) | |
| 2008 | 1,843 (31.4) | 1,972 (29.2) | |
| 2009 | 2,051 (35.0) | 2,208 (32.7) | |
| 2010 | 2,213 (37.7) | 2,404 (35.6) | |
| 2011 | 2,314 (39.4) | 2,523 (37.4) | |
| Ever enrolled | 3,197 (54.5) | 3,506 (51.9) | Fisher's exact test for greater level of overall enrollment among SHAD participants: (one-sided) p-value = 0.002. |

[a] Within-group rate dependence over the years due to enrollment in multiple years by an individual was not explicitly accounted for in this analysis. R.3.1.1 was used for this analysis.

SHAD participant and comparison populations with diagnoses from inpatient and outpatient visits to VHA facilities. In each year, a higher percentage of Project SHAD participants had at least one diagnosis in VHA records. Over the period considered, nearly 40 percent of Project SHAD participants and one-third of the comparison population had at least some record of use of the VA medical system. As with Medicare, the SHAD participants had statistically significantly higher levels as well as annual increases in use of VHA services than the comparison group (see Table 5-2). As shown in Figure 5-1, VHA usage by the two groups was initially very similar, but there was a marked increase in Project SHAD participants' use of the VA system starting in 2002. This coincides with VA's notification of SHAD veterans of their participation in Project SHAD testing and an invitation to seek additional information. By 2005, usage among SHAD veterans remained higher than that of the comparison population, but the rate of increase in use from year to year became similar in the two groups.

**TABLE 5-2** Percentage of Project SHAD Participant and Comparison Populations with Use[a] of VHA Medical Care by Year, 1999-2011

| | Received Diagnosis (%) | | |
|---|---|---|---|
| Year | Project SHAD Participants N = 5,868 | Comparison Population N = 6,753 | |
| 1999 | 612 (10.4) | 670 (9.9) | Test for differential level of VHA use between SHAD participants and comparison group was based on a logistic regression with over-dispersion[b]; (one-sided) p-value $<10^{-6}$ for additional annual increase in use. |
| 2000 | 669 (11.4) | 735 (10.9) | |
| 2001 | 752 (12.8) | 804 (11.9) | |
| 2002 | 884 (15.1) | 885 (13.1) | |
| 2003 | 1,047 (17.8) | 947 (14.0) | |
| 2004 | 1,155 (19.7) | 1,001 (14.8) | |
| 2005 | 1,146 (19.5) | 1,039 (15.4) | |
| 2006 | 1,217 (20.7) | 1,065 (15.8) | |
| 2007 | 1,227 (20.9) | 1,136 (16.8) | |
| 2008 | 1,273 (21.7) | 1,186 (17.6) | |
| 2009 | 1,336 (22.8) | 1,225 (18.1) | |
| 2010 | 1,333 (22.7) | 1,283 (19.0) | |
| 2011 | 1,395 (23.8) | 1,314 (19.5) | |
| Ever received VHA care (1997-2011) | 2,339 (39.9) | 2,235 (33.1) | Fisher's exact test for greater use of VHAD care among SHAD participants: (one-sided) p-value $<10^{-14}$. |

NOTE: VHA = Veterans Health Administration.
[a] Any diagnosis in VHA inpatient or outpatient treatment records was considered indication of use of the VHA system.
[b] Within-group rate dependence over the years due to an individual's use of services in multiple years was not explicitly accounted for in this analysis. R 3.1.1 was used for this analysis.

## OVERALL MORBIDITY

The committee used hospital days as a broad measure of significant illness in the study population. This is not a typical measure of overall morbidity, but it has been shown to predict both mortality and other hospitalizations (e.g., Wolinsky et al., 1994). No existing comorbidity index covers the range of conditions that are hypothesized to potentially be associated with SHAD participation. Some indexes (e.g., the Charlson comorbity index [Charlson et al., 1987]) are calibrated to predict 1-year mortality. Others, such as the Elixhauser comorbidity index (Elixhauser et al., 1998), are calibrated to predict medical expenses. While the committee did not believe that SHAD participation would be linked to near-term mortality among the men for whom data on health care use were available, the committee was unsure whether it would be associated with expenses. Thus, overall days of hospitalization was chosen as one sign of morbidity. When comparing those who were hospitalized through Medicare during the period 1999-2011 (see Table 5-3), Project SHAD participants had lower median hospital days per

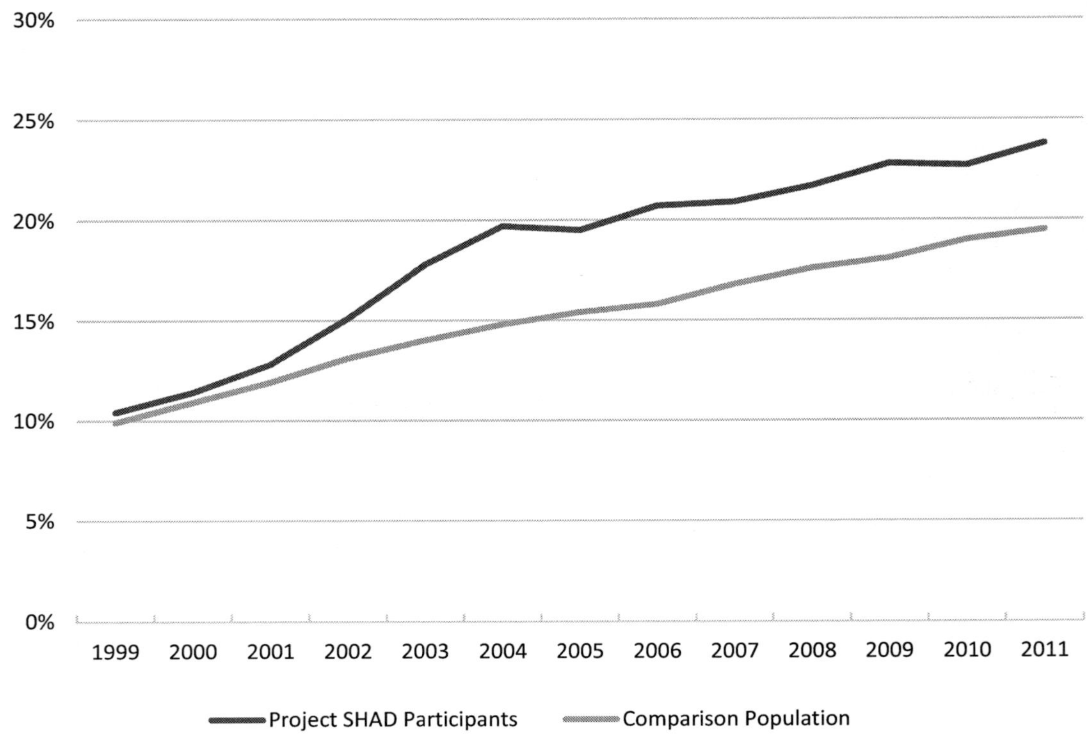


**FIGURE 5-1** Percentage of Project SHAD participant and comparison populations with any diagnosis in records of VHA medical care by year, 1999-2011.

person-year of enrollment than the comparison group, but the difference did not reach statistical significance using the Wilcoxon rank-sum test.

## CAUSE-SPECIFIC MORBIDITY

The committee also explored whether SHAD participants may have been at increased risk of illness from particular causes. Two approaches were used to look at cause-specific morbidity. One

**TABLE 5-3** Hospital Days Reflected in Medicare Fee-for-Service Claims for Project SHAD Participants and the Comparison Population Hospitalized Through Medicare, 1999-2011

| | Project SHAD Participants Ever in Medicare N = 3,197 | Comparison Population Ever Medicare N = 3,506 | Wilcoxon P-value |
|---|---|---|---|
| Hospitalized through Medicare | 1,335 (41.8%) | 1,473 (42.0%) | |
| Median hospital days per person-year of enrollment in Medicare (range), among those hospitalized | 2.00 (0.08-139.0) | 2.29 (0.08-163.0) | 0.18 |

NOTE: SAS version 9.4 was used for a two-sided Wilcoxon rank-sum test.

approach looked at the numbers of individuals receiving diagnoses within broad categories of disease that are used in the ninth revision of the *International Classification of Diseases* (ICD-9) (WHO, 2015). The morbidity analysis also examined the specific health outcomes that were identified from the review of the literature on potential health effects associated with exposure to some of the substances used in the SHAD tests. The ICD codes that correspond to the categories of illness are provided in Appendix F.

## Broad Categories of Illness

The morbidity experiences of the SHAD test participants and the members of the comparison population appeared very similar for all the diagnostic categories considered. Table 5-4 presents the numbers and percentages of the participant and comparison populations receiving a diagnosis in broad ICD-9 categories through Medicare fee-for-service during the years examined, out of the total that were ever enrolled during 1999-2011. An individual was counted as having a diagnosis in the category if there was either one inpatient diagnosis in the category, or two occurrences of an outpatient diagnosis in the category at least 1 day apart, within a 365-day period. Circulatory disease was the most common

**TABLE 5-4** SHAD Participants and Members of the Comparison Group with a Diagnosis in Broad ICD-9 Categories, Based on Claims in Medicare Fee-for-Service, 1999-2011

| | Ever Enrolled in Medicare 1999-2011 | | |
|---|---|---|---|
| Category of Illness | SHAD Participants N = 3,197 (%) | Comparison Group N = 3,506 (%) | Fisher's Exact Test Odds Ratio (95% CI) |
| Infectious disease | 403 (12.6) | 438 (12.5) | 1.01 (0.87-1.17) |
| Cancer | 546 (17.1) | 617 (17.6) | 0.96 (0.85-1.10) |
| Endocrine/metabolic disease | 1,475 (46.1) | 1,658 (47.3) | 0.95 (0.87-1.05) |
| Diseases of the blood and blood forming organs | 658 (20.6) | 732 (20.9) | 0.98 (0.87-1.11) |
| Mental disorders | 563 (17.6) | 648 (18.5) | 0.94 (0.83-1.07) |
| Nervous system and sense organs | 640 (20.0) | 772 (22.0) | 0.87 (0.79-1.00) |
| Circulatory disease | 1,622 (50.7) | 1,773 (50.6) | 1.01 (0.91-1.11) |
| Respiratory disease | 889 (27.8) | 995 (28.3) | 0.97 (0.87-1.08) |
| Digestive disease | 871 (27.2) | 942 (26.9) | 1.02 (0.91-1.14) |
| Genitourinary disease | 880 (27.5) | 966 (27.6) | 1.00 (0.90-1.11) |
| Skin disease | 315 (9.9) | 353 (10.0) | 0.98 (0.83-1.15) |
| Musculoskeletal | 861 (26.9) | 952 (27.1) | 0.99 (0.87-1.10) |
| Symptoms, signs, and abnormal clinical and laboratory findings, not elsewhere classified | 1,299 (40.6) | 1,442 (41.1) | 0.98 (0.89-1.08) |
| Injury/external causes | 1,439 (45.0) | 1,638 (46.7) | 0.93 (0.85-1.03) |
| Neurocognitive problems | 644 (20.1) | 749 (21.4) | 0.93 (0.82-1.05) |

NOTES: CI = confidence interval. See Appendix F for the ICD-9 codes that correspond to the categories of illness. An individual was counted as having a diagnosis in the category if there was either one inpatient diagnosis in the category, or two occurrences of an outpatient diagnosis in the category at least 1 day apart, within a 365-day period. R 3.1.1 was used for the Fisher's exact test and construction of confidence intervals with a two-sided alternative. No statistically significant differences were seen under the alternative of odds ratio greater than one.

diagnosis in both groups, with approximately 51 percent in each group having such a diagnosis. The proportions receiving diagnoses of other types were also comparable in the two groups. No statistically significant differences were seen. As an additional way to investigate evidence of chronic disease, the committee reviewed indicators in the Medicare records that were generated by the Chronic Condition Warehouse. These indicators mark claims related to treatment for one of 27 chronic conditions. They indicate whether "treatment for the condition appears to have taken place" using claims-based algorithms (CMS, 2015). The chronic condition data showed consistently similar percentages in the two groups (see Table 5-5).

The health experience of the SHAD participant and comparison populations also appeared very similar based on records of diagnoses from use of VHA services (see Table 5-6). As in the Medicare data, the percentages of diagnoses in various categories were similar in the SHAD veteran and comparison groups, with one exception. The percentage of SHAD veterans with an infectious disease or a musculoskeletal diagnosis was statistically significantly lower than that of the comparison population, but these differences were not in a direction of interest.

### Testing Hypotheses Regarding Specific Exposures and Health Outcomes (Morbidity)

The committee's review of literature on the agents, simulants, tracers, and decontaminants used in the SHAD tests (see Appendix C) led to the formulation of hypotheses about six of these substances, as noted in Chapter 3. It was able to test hypotheses for five of them in the evaluation of mortality in Chapter 4. In order to evaluate morbidity, it was of interest to assess the availability of information in the Medicare and VHA systems for these groups. Enrollment in fee-for-service Medicare (Part A or B) and indication of use of VHA medical care for each of these exposure groups is shown in Table 5-7. Medicare enrollment is not statistically different between in the participant and comparison groups. However, greater percentages of SHAD participants than the comparison group were seen using VHA medical care. When the committee applied an adjustment[1] to take into account the multiple tests it carried out, p-values remained statistically significant for betapropiolactone, *E. coli*, sarin, and zinc cadmium sulfide. This higher overall use of VHA health care services by those in these SHAD participant exposure subgroups is consistent with the pattern seen in Table 5-2 and Figure 5-1 of greater use of VA health care services by SHAD participants than the comparison population in general.

---

[1] The committee used False Discovery Rate (FDR) rate adjustment to take into account the multiple tests carried out. Additional detail about the application of this adjustment is provided in Appendix D.

**TABLE 5-5** Percentage of Study Subjects with a Record in the Medicare Chronic Condition Warehouse File with a Specified Diagnosis, 1999-2011

| | Number (Percent) with Diagnosis | | |
|---|---|---|---|
| Chronic Condition | Project SHAD Participants (N = 3,197) | Comparison Population (N = 3,506) | Fisher's Exact Test Odds Ratio (95% CI) |
| Acquired hypothyroidism | 196 (6.1) | 214 (6.1) | 1.00 (0.82-1.23) |
| Acute myocardial infarction | 141 (4.4) | 147 (4.2) | 1.05 (0.83-1.34) |
| Alzheimer's disease | 75 (2.3) | 73 (2.1) | 1.13 (0.80-1.59) |
| Alzheimer's disease and related disorders or senile dementia | 192 (6.0) | 203 (5.8) | 1.04 (0.84-1.28) |
| Anemia | 977 (30.6) | 1,103 (31.5) | 0.96 (0.86-1.06) |
| Asthma | 190 (5.9) | 232 (6.6) | 0.89 (0.73-1.09) |
| Atrial fibrillation | 354 (11.1) | 350 (10.0) | 1.12 (0.96-1.32) |
| Cancer of the lung | 118 (3.7) | 151 (4.3) | 0.85 (0.66-1.10) |
| Cancer of the prostate | 276 (8.6) | 284 (8.1) | 1.07 (0.90-1.28) |
| Cataract | 1,011 (31.6) | 1,140 (32.5) | 0.96 (0.86-1.07) |
| Chronic heart failure | 617 (19.3) | 676 (19.3) | 1.00 (0.89-1.13) |
| Chronic kidney disease | 539 (16.9) | 596 (17.0) | 0.99 (0.87-1.13) |
| Chronic obstructive pulmonary disease | 729 (22.8) | 841 (24.0) | 0.94 (0.83-1.05) |
| Colorectal cancer | 69 (2.2) | 95 (2.7) | 0.79 (0.57-1.10) |
| Depression | 435 (13.6) | 488 (13.9) | 0.97 (0.85-1.12) |
| Diabetes | 921 (28.8) | 1,020 (29.1) | 0.99 (0.89-1.10) |
| Glaucoma | 300 (9.4) | 358 (10.2) | 0.91 (0.77-1.07) |
| Hip fracture | 38 (1.2) | 51 (1.5) | 0.81 (0.52-1.27) |
| Hyperlipidemia | 1,640 (51.3) | 1,803 (51.4) | 0.99 (0.90-1.10) |
| Hyperplasia, benign prostatic | 704 (22.0) | 806 (23.0) | 0.95 (0.84-1.06) |
| Hypertension | 1,815 (56.8) | 2,004 (57.2) | 0.98 (0.89-1.09) |
| Ischemic heart disease | 1,200 (37.5) | 1,295 (36.9) | 1.03 (0.93-1.13) |
| Osteoporosis | 88 (2.8) | 99 (2.8) | 0.97 (0.72-1.32) |
| Rheumatoid arthritis/ osteoarthritis | 758 (23.7) | 865 (24.7) | 0.95 (0.85-1.06) |
| Stroke/transient ischemic attack | 282 (8.8) | 341 (9.7) | 0.90 (0.76-1.06) |

NOTES: CI = confidence interval. Algorithms used to define the chronic conditions are available from the Chronic Conditions Data Warehouse (CMS, 2015). R 3.1.1 was used for the Fisher's exact test and construction of confidence intervals with a two-sided alternative. No statistically significant differences were seen between the SHAD participant group and the comparison group under the alternative of odds ratio greater than 1.

**TABLE 5-6** SHAD Participant and Comparison Populations with Diagnoses in Broad ICD-9 Categories from Use of VHA Inpatient or Outpatient Services, 1997-2011

| | Number (%) with Diagnosis | | |
|---|---|---|---|
| Diagnosis Category | Project SHAD Participants N = 2,339 | Comparison Population N = 2,235 | Fisher's Exact Test Odds Ratio (95% CI) |
| Infectious disease | 682 (29.2) | 720 (32.2) | **0.87** (0.76-0.98) |
| Cancer | 979 (41.9) | 899 (40.2) | 1.07 (0.95-1.21) |
| Endocrine/metabolic disease | 1,740 (74.4) | 1,708 (76.4) | 0.90 (0.78-1.03) |
| Diseases of the blood and blood forming organs | 475 (20.3) | 488 (21.8) | 0.91 (0.79-1.05) |
| Mental disorders | 1,281 (54.8) | 1,257 (56.2) | 0.94 (0.84-1.06) |
| Nervous system and sense organs | 1,598 (68.3) | 1,559 (69.8) | 0.94 (0.82-1.06) |
| Circulatory disease | 1,791 (76.6) | 1,730 (77.4) | 0.95 (0.83-1.10) |
| Respiratory disease | 1,163 (49.7) | 1,118 (50.0) | 0.99 (0.88-1.11) |
| Digestive disease | 1,285 (54.9) | 1,256 (56.2) | 0.95 (0.84-1.07) |
| Genitourinary disease | 1,090 (46.6) | 1,064 (47.6) | 0.96 (0.85-1.08) |
| Skin disease | 1,043 (44.6) | 956 (42.8) | 1.08 (0.96-1.21) |
| Musculoskeletal | 1,412 (60.4) | 1,431 (64.0) | **0.86** (0.76-0.97) |
| Symptoms, signs, and abnormal clinical and laboratory findings, not elsewhere classified | 1,627 (69.6) | 1,578 (70.6) | 0.95 (0.84-1.08) |
| Injury/external causes | 2,246 (96.0) | 2,126 (95.1) | 1.24 (0.92-1.66) |
| Neurocognitive problems | 1,301 (55.6) | 1,282 (57.4) | 0.93 (0.83-1.05) |

NOTES: CI = confidence interval. See Appendix F for the ICD-9 codes that correspond to the categories of illness. An individual was counted as having a diagnosis in the category if there was either one inpatient diagnosis in the category, or two occurrences of an outpatient diagnosis in the category at least 1 day apart, within a 365-day period. R 3.1.1 was used for Fisher's exact tests and construction of confidence intervals with a two-sided alternative. No statistically significant differences were seen between the SHAD participant group and the comparison group under the alternative of odds ratio greater than 1.

## All-Cause Morbidity for Selected Exposures

As with the complete study population, the committee used median Medicare hospital days per person-year of enrollment as a means to assess significant illness in the groups exposed to selected substances and their comparison groups (see Table 5-8). Median hospital days per person-year of enrollment were not statistically different between Project SHAD participants in the exposure groups and the comparison groups, except in the case of betapropiolactone where the median hospital days per person-year of enrollment were lower among those in the SHAD tests.

**TABLE 5-7** Percentage of SHAD Participants with Specified Exposures and Their Comparison Groups Who Were Enrolled in Fee-for-Service Medicare (1999-2011) or Used[a] VHA Medical Care (1997-2011)

| Exposure and Data Source | Project SHAD Participants | Comparison Population | Fisher's Exact Test Odds Ratio (95% CI) | P-value |
|---|---|---|---|---|
| *Coxiella burnetii* | | | | |
| N | 141 | 212 | | |
| Medicare | 60.3% | 62.7% | 0.90 (0.57-1.43) | 0.7181 |
| VHA | 41.8% | 30.7% | **1.62 (1.02-2.60)** | **0.02082** |
| Betapropiolactone | | | | |
| N | 595 | 607 | | |
| Medicare | 62.2% | 57.8% | 1.20 (0.95-1.52) | 0.06894 |
| VHA | 40.7% | 30.5% | **1.56 (1.22-2.00)** | **0.00014**[b] |
| *Escherichia coli* | | | | |
| N | 141 | 228 | | |
| Medicare | 55.3% | 54.4% | 1.04 (0.67-1.62) | 0.4735 |
| VHA | 46.8% | 34.2% | **1.69 (1.08-2.66)** | **0.01084**[b] |
| Sarin | | | | |
| N | 129 | 197 | | |
| Medicare | 65.1% | 60.4% | 1.22 (0.75-2.00) | 0.2296 |
| VHA | 45.0% | 32.5% | **1.69 (1.05-2.75)** | **0.01561**[b] |
| Zinc cadmium sulfide | | | | |
| N | 681 | 773 | | |
| Medicare | 60.9% | 59.1% | 1.08 (0.87-1.34) | 0.2569 |
| VHA | 42.4% | 32.5% | **1.53 (1.23-1.91)** | **5.443e-5**[b] |

NOTES: CI = confidence interval; VHA = Veterans Health Administration. R.3.1 was used for the Fisher's exact test and construction of confidence intervals with a two-sided alternative.

[a] Any diagnosis in VHA inpatient or outpatient treatment records was considered indication of use of the VHA system.

[b] P-values under the alternative of odds ratio greater than 1 were adjusted for a 5 percent false discovery rate (FDR) taking into account 10 tests; those with a [b] remained statistically significant at the 5 percent FDR level.

## Morbidity from Health Outcomes with a Hypothesized Association with Certain SHAD Test Exposures

The committee also examined in both Medicare and VHA data diagnoses for the specific health outcomes that the committee concluded were suggested by the scientific literature to be a possible effect from certain exposures (see Table 3-1). Counts of those SHAD veterans potentially exposed to these substances who were diagnosed with the outcomes in Medicare or VHA records are presented in Table 5-9. Criteria for counting a diagnosis are shown in the table's notes.

**TABLE 5-8** Hospital Days Reflected in Medicare Fee-for-Service Claims for Project SHAD Participants with Specified Exposures and Comparison Groups Hospitalized Through Medicare, 1999-2011

| Exposure | Project SHAD Participants | Comparison Group | Wilcoxon Rank Sum Test P-value |
|---|---|---|---|
| *Coxiella burnetii* | | | |
| Number enrolled in Medicare | 85 | 133 | |
| Hospitalized through Medicare | 45 (52.9%) | 62 (46.6%) | |
| Median hospital days per person-year of enrollment in Medicare (range), among hospitalized | 1.78 (0.22-24.75) | 1.97 (0.17-46.0) | 0.76 |
| Betapropiolactone | | | |
| Number enrolled in Medicare | 370 | 351 | |
| Hospitalized through Medicare | 162 (46.1%) | 154 (41.6%) | |
| Median hospital days per person-year of enrollment in Medicare (range), among hospitalized | 1.70 (0.15-48.8) | 2.75 (0.15-75.0) | **0.03** |
| *Escherichia coli* | | | |
| Number enrolled in Medicare | 78 | 124 | |
| Hospitalized through Medicare | 32 (41.0%) | 56 (45.2%) | |
| Median hospital days per person-year of enrollment in Medicare (range), among hospitalized | 2.00 (0.33-47.4) | 2.34 (0.08-75.17) | 0.66 |
| Sarin | | | |
| Number enrolled in Medicare | 84 | 119 | |
| Hospitalized through Medicare | 34 (40.5%) | 58 (48.7%) | |
| Median hospital days per person-year of enrollment in Medicare (range), among hospitalized | 1.85 (0.23-42.0) | 1.50 (0.17-46.0) | 0.89 |
| Zinc cadmium sulfide | | | |
| Number enrolled in Medicare | 415 | 457 | |
| Hospitalized through Medicare | 190 (45.8%) | 199 (43.5%) | |
| Median hospital days per person-year of enrollment in Medicare (range), among hospitalized | 1.86 (0.15-47.4) | 2.40 (0.08-75.17) | 0.09 |

NOTE: SAS version 9.4 was used for a two-sided Wilcoxon rank-sum test.

Taking into account the numbers of people enrolled in Medicare or seeking care through VHA, the SHAD veterans with exposures to *C. burnetii*, betapriopiolactone, or zinc cadmium sulfide had generally similar percentages with diagnoses for the hypothesized illnesses as those in the comparison groups. In addition, the percentages with diagnoses in the Medicare and VHA data were similar. In the group of SHAD veterans exposed to *E. coli*, a few cases of irritable bowel syndrome were seen in Medicare records (too few to allow reporting of a specific number), but no cases were seen in the VHA records. In the comparison group for this exposure no diagnoses for irritable bowel syndrome were seen in either the Medicare or VHA records. A smaller percentage of the SHAD veterans than the comparison group had diagnoses potentially associated with exposure to sarin in the Medicare data, but the pattern was reversed in the VHA data, with a greater percentage of the SHAD veterans than the comparison group having diagnoses of interest. No statistically significant differences were seen in these comparisons.

**TABLE 5-9** SHAD Participant and Comparison Groups with Specified Exposures and Diagnoses of Interest in Medicare Fee-for-Service Enrollees (1999-2011) and VHA Users (1997-2011)

| Exposure | Project SHAD Participants | Comparison Group | Fisher's Exact Test Odds Ratio (95% CI) |
|---|---|---|---|
| *Coxiella burnetii* | | | |
| Number with any diagnosis of interest[a] in Medicare records | ≤10 | 13 | NR (0.27-2.35) |
| Number enrolled in Medicare | 85 | 133 | |
| Percent of Medicare enrollees with diagnosis of interest | NR | 10% | |
| Number with any diagnosis of interest in VHA records | ≤10 | ≤10 | 1.23 (0.34-4.40) |
| Number with any diagnosis in VHA | 59 | 71 | |
| Percent of the VHA users with diagnosis of interest | NR | NR | |
| Betapropiolactone | | | |
| Number with any cancer in Medicare records | 59 | 52 | 1.09 (0.71-1.67) |
| Number enrolled in Medicare | 370 | 351 | |
| Percent of Medicare enrollees with diagnosis of interest | 16% | 15% | |
| Number with any cancer in VHA records | 53 | 45 | 0.87 (0.54-1.41) |
| Number with any diagnosis in VHA | 242 | 185 | |
| Percent of the VHA users with diagnosis of interest | 22% | 24% | |
| *Escherichia coli* | | | |
| Number with irritable bowel syndrome in Medicare records | ≤10 | 0 | NR (0.28-2.35) |
| Number enrolled in Medicare | 78 | 124 | |
| Percent of Medicare enrollees with diagnosis of interest | NR | 0 | |
| Number with irritable bowel syndrome in the VHA records | 0 | 0 | |
| Number with any diagnosis in VHA | 66 | 78 | |
| Percent of the VHA users with diagnosis | 0 | 0 | |

| Exposure | Project SHAD Participants | Comparison Group | Fisher's Exact Test Odds Ratio (95% CI) |
|---|---|---|---|
| of interest | | | |
| **Sarin** | | | |
| Number with any diagnosis of interest[b] in Medicare records | 19 | 34 | 0.73 (0.36-1.46) |
| Number enrolled in Medicare | 84 | 119 | |
| Percent of Medicare enrollees with diagnosis of interest | 23% | 29% | |
| Number with any diagnosis of interest in the VHA records | 42 | 42 | 1.37 (0.59-3.22) |
| Number with any diagnosis in VHA | 58 | 64 | |
| Percent of the VHA users with diagnosis of interest | 72% | 65% | |
| **Zinc cadmium sulfide** | | | |
| Number with any diagnosis of interest[c] in Medicare records | 61 | 61 | 1.12 (0.75-1.67) |
| Number enrolled in Medicare | 415 | 457 | |
| Percent of Medicare enrollees with diagnosis of interest | 15% | 13% | |
| Number with any diagnosis of interest in the VHA records | 42 | 43 | 0.82 (0.50-1.34) |
| Number with any diagnosis in VHA | 289 | 289 | |
| Percent of VHA users with diagnosis of interest | 15% | 17% | |

NOTES: CI = confidence interval; NR = not reported, cell size ≤10 could be back-calculated; VHA = Veterans Health Administration.
Medicare data: Counts represent individuals assigned a diagnostic code for the disease or condition of interest in Medicare fee-for-service records for the period 1999-2011. Diagnostic codes for these conditions are listed in Appendix F. For inpatient data, any record with the requisite code was counted. For outpatient data, a diagnosis was counted if it had at least two occurrences at least 1 day apart, within a 365-day period.
VHA data: Counts represent individuals assigned a diagnostic code for the disease or condition of interest in VHA records for the period 1997-2011. Diagnostic codes for these conditions are listed in Appendix F. For inpatient data, any record with the requisite code was counted. For outpatient data, a diagnosis was counted if it had at least two occurrences at least 1 day apart, within a 365-day period. R 3.1.1 was used for the Fisher's exact tests and construction of confidence intervals with a two-sided alternative. Fisher's exact tests were also conducted under the alternative odds ratio greater than 1; none of the tests was significant at the nominal level 0.05 before FDR correction.
[a] Diagnosis of endocarditis, fatigue, chronic hepatitis, osteomyelitis, or vascular infection.
[b] Diagnosis of central or peripheral system neurological effects, hearing loss, or psychological symptoms.
[c] Diagnosis of lung cancer or chronic kidney disease.

## REFERENCES

Charlson, M. E., P. Pompei, K. L. Ales, and C. R. MacKenzie. 1987. A new method of classifying prognostic comorbidity in longitudinal studies: Development and validation. *Journal of Chronic Diseases* 40:373-383.

CMS (Centers for Medicare & Medicaid Services). 2015. *Chronic conditions data warehouse: Condition categories.* https://www.ccwdata.org/web/guest/condition-categories (accessed October 23, 2015).

Elixhauser, A., C. Steiner, D. R. Harris, and R. M Coffey. 1998. Comorbidity measures for use with administrative data. *Medical Care* 36(1):8-27.

WHO (World Health Organization). 2015. *International Classification of Diseases (ICD).* http://www.who.int/classifications/icd/en (accessed August 4, 2015).

Wolinsky, F. D., S. D. Culler, C. M. Callahan, and R. J. Johnson. 1994. Hospital resource consumption among older adults: A prospective analysis of episodes, length of stay, and charges over a seven-year period. *Journal of Gerontology* 49:S240-S252.

# 6

# Discussion

During the 1960s, nearly 5,900 members of the armed forces were present during the Shipboard Hazard and Defense tests—Project SHAD—that were conducted to assess vulnerabilities to and defenses against chemical and biological warfare at sea. The analysis described in this report was carried out to assess whether these men have been at increased risk for adverse health outcomes because of their participation in Project SHAD. This chapter provides a summary and interpretation of the findings of the analysis of the second Institute of Medicine (IOM) review of health outcomes among SHAD veterans, and describes its strengths and weaknesses for answering the questions posed.

## FINDINGS ON MORTALITY

The committee examined the mortality data for the study population using three approaches: (1) The entire Project SHAD participant population was compared to the total population that served on comparison vessels and in comparison air and ground units. (2) Exposure-specific comparisons were made between SHAD participants and comparison groups to test hypotheses suggested by the scientific literature regarding health risks. (3) Additional exploratory analyses were carried out for groups established based upon the substance(s) used in the tests in which they participated, or the particular combination of substances to which they were exposed. The rationale for these groupings is described in Chapter 3.

The committee carried out multiple statistical tests in its examination of mortality differences in the groups described. Testing a large number of exposure-outcome associations increases the chance of reporting spurious associations. As a final step in the interpretation of its results, the committee applied statistical adjustments to account for the multiple comparisons in its analysis.

### Overall Mortality

The Project SHAD participants and the comparison group were similar in terms of age, race where known, and proportions who were officers or enlisted personnel (see Table 4-1). Their survival experience was also similar, with no statistically significant difference in all-cause mortality (see Table 4-3). No statistically significant increases in hazard for Project SHAD participants were seen when cause-specific mortality was examined.

## Hypotheses Regarding Specific Exposures and Causes of Death

The committee paid particular attention to those Project SHAD test veterans who had been in tests that included the use of *Coxiella burnetii*, betapropiolactone (BPL), *Escherichia coli* (*E. coli*), sarin, or zinc cadmium sulfide because its review of the scientific literature (described in Appendix C) suggested the possibility that people exposed to these substances might be at increased risk for specific adverse health effects.[1] The analysis of these hypotheses examined both all-cause mortality in the groups exposed to these substances and mortality from specific causes.

There were no significant differences between the exposed and comparison groups for all-cause mortality, either for the groups as a whole, or when officers and enlisted personnel were examined separately. In examining cause-specific mortality, the committee found no deaths attributed to most of the hypothesized health effects among either the participant or comparison groups (see Table 4-7). Deaths from cancer in general and lung cancer in particular could be analyzed in more detail. The hazard ratio for mortality from cancer was not statistically different in those exposed to BPL compared to the appropriate comparison units. The SHAD veterans who were exposed to zinc cadmium sulfide had a slight excess in lung cancer deaths that did not reach statistical significance (see Table 4-8). For both BPL and zinc cadmium sulfide exposure groups, no difference was found between the SHAD veterans and the comparison groups when the enlisted group was examined separately.

The committee also examined the effect of the number of opportunities for exposure to these substances. No association with increasing mortality from cancer was observed in those with more potential exposure to BPL or zinc cadmium sulfide (see Table 4-9).

## Exploratory Analyses of Mortality

The committee sought to be particularly thorough in its analyses and open to the potential for findings that were not suggested by its review of the literature. The SHAD tests involved multiple experiences which could for some participants have included aspects not captured by the reports from the Department of Defense (DoD) of substances used in the tests. The committee therefore also examined mortality in six additional groups. These groupings were defined as (1) exposure to any biological test substance; (2) exposure to any chemical test substance (except trioctyl phosphate [TOF]); (3) exposure to any decontaminant; (4) exposure to TOF, which was used only in Test 69-10; (5) service on the light tugs or as Project SHAD staff on the USS *Granville S. Hall*, and (6) service on the USS *George Eastman*.

There were no overall differences in survival when the six groups were compared with their respective comparison groups, or when stratified by rank (officer or enlisted) (see Table 4-11). No association with increasing mortality was seen with increasing exposure to "any biological substance," "any chemical substance," or "any decontaminant" in the groups for

---

[1] The committee's review of the literature also generated hypotheses of long-term effects from exposure to Staphylococcal enterotoxin type B, but a roster of individuals participating in this test was not available to test the hypotheses.

which there was sufficient sample size and variability in number of exposures to evaluate (see Table 4-12).[2]

Analysis of cause-specific mortality for the groups of participants exposed to "any biological substance," "any chemical substance," "any decontaminant," and the tugs and Project SHAD technical staff found that the groups did not show significantly increased mortality from that of their comparison groups. The only statistically significant result suggesting increased risk for a Project SHAD participant group was an increase in the hazard ratio for heart disease among the crew of the USS *George Eastman*. Ischemic heart disease mortality contributed the greater portion to this increased hazard ratio, but was not itself statistically different in between SHAD participants and the comparison group. When the committee applied a statistical adjustment to take into account the multiple comparisons in the analysis of cause-specific mortality within the crew of the *George Eastman*, the result no longer attained statistical significance.

### Interpretation of the Mortality Results

The previous IOM (2007) study of SHAD veterans (referred to as SHAD I) did not observe statistically significant differences in all-cause mortality between participants and the comparison group for the total study population. The results of the present study, with an additional 7 years of mortality follow-up, are similar. The SHAD I study found an elevation in heart disease mortality for SHAD veterans overall, and supplementary analyses following the SHAD I study (IOM, 2008) observed an elevated all-cause mortality risk for the crew of the USS *George Eastman.* The USS *George Eastman* was a ship specially outfitted for participation in SHAD testing and was involved in multiple tests. In the current study, an increase in heart disease risk was seen only for the crew of the USS *George Eastman*. However, it is important not to over-interpret the elevated heart disease risk seen in the current study, as an adjustment for the multiple testing carried out indicates the likelihood that this could have resulted from chance alone.

## FINDINGS ON MORBIDITY

Morbidity in the study population was evaluated using records from automated databases from Medicare and the Veterans Health Administration (VHA). The Medicare data reflect claims for fee-for-service hospital or outpatient care during the period 1999-2011. Overall, 55 percent of the SHAD participants and 52 percent of the comparison population were enrolled in Medicare (Parts A or B) for some of this time. For most years, the SHAD test participants had slightly higher Medicare enrollment than the comparison population (see Table 5-1), which may reflect that the SHAD veterans were slightly older than the comparison population (see Table 4-1).

VHA records covered inpatient and outpatient care during the period 1997-2011. Up to 40 percent of Project SHAD participants and a third of the comparison population had diagnoses recorded; use of VHA services was consistently higher among SHAD veterans than the comparison population during the time examined (see Table 5-2). The committee noted that the proportionally greater use of VHA by Project SHAD participants became more marked starting in 2002 when the Department of Veterans Affairs (VA) sent letters to SHAD veterans informing them of their participation in SHAD tests and making available health evaluations at VA (see

---

[2] See Box 3-1 for a list of the test substances covered by each of these groups.

Figure 5-1). It seems plausible that this notification contributed to an increased use of VHA services by SHAD veterans. Other factors, including the possibility that the SHAD veteran population was consistently less healthy and sought care preferentially through VHA, may also have contributed but are harder to isolate.

The committee used two approaches to assessing morbidity. Consistent with the analysis of mortality, the entire Project SHAD participant population was compared to the total population that served on vessels and in airborne and ground units that were selected for the comparison population. In addition, exposure-specific comparisons were made between SHAD participants and the corresponding comparison groups to test hypotheses suggested by the scientific literature regarding health risks. Time and resources did not permit analysis of morbidity for the special exposure groups for which further exploratory mortality analyses were conducted. As with mortality, statistical adjustments for the multiple testing carried out were applied to the findings.

Overall, or all-cause, morbidity was evaluated using median hospital days per person-year of enrollment among Medicare enrollees hospitalized during the study period. Hospital days provide a measure of relatively significant illness of all kinds. Cause-specific morbidity was evaluating by looking at numbers of people with diagnoses in Medicare or VHA records. Broad categories from the ninth revision of the *International Classification of Diseases* (ICD-9) (WHO, 2015) were used for analyses of the population as a whole, and specific diagnoses were used in the analyses that focused on the health outcomes hypothesized for the substances of interest (see Table 3-1).

### Overall Morbidity

Roughly 42 percent of both Project SHAD participant and comparison groups who had been enrolled in Medicare during the study period had a hospitalization during that time. Median hospital days per person-year of enrollment among those hospitalized was slightly lower among Project SHAD participants than the comparison group, but the difference was not statistically significant (see Table 5-3).

Cause-specific morbidity was examined using diagnoses from both Medicare and VHA records. The analysis of Medicare data considered broad ICD-9 categories of disease (see Table 5-4) as well as chronic conditions flagged by Medicare's Chronic Condition Warehouse (CCW) (see Table 5-5). The CCW files indicate whether "treatment for the condition appears to have taken place" using claims-based algorithms (CMS, 2015).

For both broad categories of illness and specific chronic conditions, no statistically significant differences were seen between the Project SHAD participant and comparison groups.

Similarly, the percentages of those with diagnoses within major categories of illness in VA records were largely the same in the overall SHAD participant and comparison populations. The VA data provide different information than the Medicare data because a "true" number of people in the study who might have been able to use the VA system (for administrative, geographic, or other reasons) is not known. Instead, the denominator used in Table 5-6 is that of people who have sought care in VA in any of the years noted. The percentages of those with diagnoses are higher than in Medicare, probably because these are percentages of those seeking health care rather than of a general veteran population.

### Hypotheses Regarding Specific Exposures and Morbidity

As noted above, the committee's review of the scientific literature suggested the possibility that people exposed to *C. burnetii*, BPL, *E. coli*, sarin, or zinc cadmium sulfide might be at increased risk for certain adverse health effects. The hypotheses were tested by examining both overall morbidity and morbidity from the specific adverse health effects in the groups exposed to these substances.

Fifty-five to 65 percent of participants in the exposure and comparison groups were enrolled in Medicare during the period in question. From the VHA data it was seen that 40 percent to 47 percent of the SHAD veterans in these exposure groups had a diagnosis recorded in the VHA data and thus were known to have used the VHA system. Only 30 to 34 percent of those in the comparison groups were known to use the VHA system (see Table 5-7). The differences in use of VHA health care for most of these exposure groups was statistically significantly higher among the SHAD participants than for the comparison groups, even after correction for multiple testing. This result was consistent with heavier use of VHA health care seen for the Project SHAD participant group as a whole. As noted earlier, this higher level of use may have resulted from the letters of notification sent to Project SHAD participants that invited them to have a health assessment at VA. Of those enrolled in Medicare, 41 to 53 percent were hospitalized during the study period. Among those hospitalized, median hospital days per person-year of enrollment among the SHAD veterans in the exposure groups were not statistically greater than their comparison groups (see Table 5-8).

Finally, the committee used both Medicare and VHA data to assess whether the specific health outcomes hypothesized were observed more frequently in the SHAD veterans in these exposure groups than in the comparison groups. On the basis of the percentages of those enrolled in Medicare or who had used the VHA system who had a diagnosis of interest, the SHAD veterans and their comparison groups had similar results (see Table 5-9). Odds ratios for the counts showed no statistically significant differences.

### Interpretation of Morbidity Results

The current study did not identify consistent differences in morbidity between Project SHAD participants and the comparison group for the study population as a whole or for specific exposure groups. The committee notes that the SHAD I study analyzed responses to a 2004 health survey that indicated worse health among the surviving SHAD veterans than the comparison group. However, the SHAD I health survey also collected reports of hospitalizations and found no significant differences, which is consistent with the finding of the current study.

## THE STUDY'S STRENGTHS AND WEAKNESSES

### Strengths of the Study

The current study benefited from a considerable investment of effort during the first IOM study (IOM, 2007) to establish and validate the cohort of Project SHAD test participants from ship logs and diaries. Except for the few cases where ship logs or rosters were not available,[3] the

---

[3] Rosters were not available for the tug boats that participated in tests other than Shady Grove.

researchers were largely able to identify personnel sufficiently for follow-up. The SHAD I report (IOM, 2007) noted that, except for the personnel from Test 69-10, less than 6 percent of the study population lacked social security numbers, permitting fairly complete follow up.

The study also benefited from the input of SHAD veterans. At the start of this second SHAD study, the committee held two public meetings at which veterans were invited to share their experiences. At the second meeting, panels of men who had been part of the Project SHAD Technical Staff, the Copper Head test, and Test 69-10 recounted some of their memories of the testing and answered committee member questions (see Appendix B). These interactions with SHAD veterans helped the committee to better understand the context of the tests and the experience of those who had been present.

The study's cohort design was strengthened by the use of a comparison group selected to be as similar as possible to the group with the exposure under study. In contrast to studies in which military personnel are compared to civilians, or deployed service members to the non-deployed, this study had the advantage of comparing groups who were deployed at the same time and in similar areas.

Another strength of this study is the length of follow up. By the end of the study follow-up period, December 31, 2011, nearly 50 years had elapsed since the earliest SHAD tests in 1963, and 42 years since the final tests in 1969. Because of this lengthy follow-up period, the study had an opportunity to assess the mortality experience of the study population across a broad range of causes of death, including those that appear later in life. Similarly, the long follow-up period made it feasible to turn to Medicare data to examine morbidity.

The availability of information on cause of death from the National Death Index for deaths from 1979 forward was another factor in making it possible to conduct a range of mortality analyses. The current study added to the mortality information available in SHAD I by also seeking death certificates for members of the study population who died before 1979. As described in Chapter 3 and Appendix D, nearly 200 additional death certificates were obtained through requests to individual states.

As previously noted, the SHAD I study relied on a survey to solicit reports from the surviving members of the study population on their health. Although such surveys make it possible to assess a broad range of indicators of health status, they depend for their validity on the accuracy and completeness of reporting by the respondents and on the response rate. They also require direct contact with each surviving member of the study population. Using Medicare and VHA databases made it possible to obtain highly detailed information on diagnoses made by medical professionals over multiple years for veterans who received care during the period for which records were obtained. Using these sources increases the quality of information for all included in this study and protects against the effects of differential mortality, recall bias, confusion about medical terminology, and health-related causes of non-response (e.g., persons who are sicker typically have lower response rates than those who are healthier, but they are more likely to appear in Medicare claims data because they receive more care).

Given the broad range of potential health outcomes, the study also benefited from the committee's review of the literature concerning the agents, simulants, decontaminants and tracers used in the tests to formulate hypotheses to test in the study.

## Weaknesses of the Study

Exposure misclassification has been referred to as "the Achilles' heel" of environmental epidemiology. In this study the committee felt it was able to refine the representations of exposure by taking into account the numbers of trials in which SHAD veterans had the opportunity to be exposed to a given test substance. However, this remains an indirect form of exposure assessment. Data were not available to determine the dose of a substance received by individual participants or, for most tests, the environmental concentrations of the test substances to which service members were exposed. Requests from the committee for declassification of such information from these tests were not approved by DoD.

Knowledge of one's exposure status has the potential to bias the detection of the outcomes of interest because a person who considers himself exposed may be more likely to seek health care or recall health conditions than a person who does not consider himself exposed. In 2002, VA (2002) began notifying SHAD veterans that they had been part of the SHAD test program and that they could seek health assessments from VA. Since then, the SHAD participants have had time to seek health care and receive diagnoses that veterans in the comparison population may not have sought.

The SHAD tests took place during the Vietnam era; therefore both SHAD participants and the members of the comparison population may also have had service that makes them eligible for disability claims for certain conditions that VA has declared are presumptively related to Agent Orange exposure (VA, 2015). Since the early 1990s, growing numbers of Vietnam veterans have been deemed to have service-related conditions related to Agent Orange exposure. As of January 2015, more than a dozen medical conditions are included (e.g., diabetes, ischemic heart disease, lung cancer, prostate cancer, and Parkinson's disease). Eligibility has also been expanded to include not only personnel who served as ground troops in Vietnam, but also (on a case-by-case basis) the "blue-water" Navy service members as well as some veterans with service in Korea or Thailand (VA, 2015).

A potential weakness of the study is an inability to tell whether participant and control populations had similar levels of exposure to service in Vietnam. In addition to potential exposure to Agent Orange, traumatic experience increases risks to mental and physical health (e.g., Boscarino, 2008). The extent to which the two groups differ on Vietnam-related service is not known, but VA records indicate similar percentages of Vietnam service among the SHAD participants (17.4 percent) and the comparison population (18.4 percent) that had filed a disability claim (see Table 4-1).

Another aspect of the analysis is that while mortality data were available for the entire period since the time of the testing, morbidity data were available only for the period beginning in the late 1990s. Thus, health effects arising soon after exposure could be detected in these analyses only if they led to higher mortality or highly persistent morbidity.

Finally, the committee's use of hypotheses generated from the literature provided some focus for the analyses, but in assessing the health status of SHAD participants and the comparison groups for various categories of exposures the committee carried out many statistical tests, increasing the likelihood that statistically significant associations could arise by chance. In some cases the exposure groups were of modest size, which could make it difficult to ascertain any true subtle differences in either mortality or morbidity.

## ANALYTICAL CHALLENGES

This analysis proved to be challenging for several reasons. First, the Medicare and VHA data can be broadly interpreted as indications of health by their reflection of diagnoses that lead to health care use. The Medicare data for enrollees over age 65 can be interpreted as providing population-based measures; however, the VHA data generally cannot be because of the variable criteria associated with eligibility for these services and the decision-making process associated with their use. Second, at no time was the entire Project SHAD participant cohort eligible for Medicare. Thus, the committee's analysis had to focus on the morbidity of the oldest veterans, who were also the oldest at the time of the testing. Finally, the data themselves are quite complex. Once enrolled in Medicare, each person will have one annual enrollment record but will have variable numbers of physician, hospital, and medication records that contain information about diagnoses. These records need to be combined into specific yes/no variables such as "diagnosis of neurological disorder." With Medicare enrollment beginning at age 65, the identified cases reflect a combination of existing (prevalent) disease at age 65 and new (incident) disease diagnosed after age 65. These features of the data on the timing of health outcomes, combined with the challenges associated with assessing exposure, resulted in a study with many analytical complexities.

## OTHER CONCERNS

### Continued Classification of the Test Documents

As noted in Chapter 1, the committee requested declassification of additional data pertaining to the tests and exposures. Ultimately, no additional materials were declassified and made available to the committee, out of concern that vulnerabilities that might have been identified by the SHAD testing could still be relevant despite turnover in the naval fleet. The committee notes that the information that remains classified might have informed understanding of the range of concentrations of test substances to which participants might have been exposed, but information about the location of personnel on the vessels during the tests and the doses they may have received would still have been absent. The statistical analyses would still be based on comparing exposure groups. As a result, the committee does not expect that access to the classified information would have altered the findings of the analysis.

### Human Health and Ethics

In the decades that have passed since the SHAD testing, views on both workplace safety and the inclusion of humans (intentionally or not) in experimental testing have undergone a major evolution and emphasize the importance of informing workers (including military service personnel) of the chemicals (and potential health risk) they may be exposed to. The approximately 5,900 military personnel reported to have been included in the Project SHAD testing were not unknowingly participating in human-subjects research, but because of the security around the testing, service personnel were not necessarily aware of the purposes of the testing and the agents being used. Review of the test plans and descriptions of the tests show that the intent of the program was to evaluate operational characteristics of ships and protective and dissemination equipment as well as the behavior of test agents in marine environments.

While it is evident that the intent of SHAD was not to evaluate the health impact of exposure to the substances used in the tests, animals were used in some of the tests and reportedly exposed to deadly or dangerous agents. In a few tests to evaluate personal protective equipment (e.g., Autumn Gold, DTC 69-10, Copper Head), samples such as gargle samples or chemical dosimeters on clothing were collected from service members. The secrecy surrounding the tests, the use of animal testing, and the human biological samples obtained could have led to a perception that the personnel on the tests were either purposefully or inadvertently exposed to agents with the potential for human health risk.

Although the committee was cognizant of the questions raised by veterans and others about the ethics and legality of the SHAD testing, it was not charged with reviewing the merits of the program. Its focus had to be on the scientific question of whether test participation is associated with adverse long-term health effects.

## CONCLUSIONS

Epidemiological studies such as this investigation of health outcomes among veterans of the SHAD tests are complex undertakings requiring substantial time and resources. The committee invested considerable effort in learning about the SHAD tests and in formulating its approaches to data analysis. In the numerous analyses of both the full study population and of several subgroups, the only finding of a seemingly higher risk—of heart disease mortality among the 356 men who served on the USS *George Eastman*—did not attain statistical significance after adjustments for the multiple tests carried out on this group. The vast majority of the analyses showed no evidence of different health outcomes among SHAD veterans relative to the comparison group. The committee recognizes that with the limitations of epidemiological studies these negative findings cannot unequivocally rule out some potential effect from the SHAD testing. However, within the limits of the data available to the committee, the results of the analyses provide no evidence that the health of SHAD veterans overall or those in the exposure groups is significantly different from that of similar veterans who did not participate in these tests.

## REFERENCES

Boscarino, J. A. 2008. A prospective study of PTSD and early-age heart disease mortality among Vietnam veterans: Implications for surveillance and prevention. *Psychosomatic Medicine* 70:668-676.

CMS (Centers for Medicare & Medicaid Services). 2015. *Chronic conditions data warehouse.* https://www.ccwdata.org/web/guest/condition-categories (accessed October 23, 2015).

IOM (Institute of Medicine). 2007. *Long-term health effects of participation in Project SHAD (Shipboard Hazard and Defense).* Washington, DC: The National Academies Press.

IOM. 2008. *Response to 15 February 2008 letter from Congressmen Mike Thompson and Dennis Rehberg.* http://iom.nationalacademies.org/~/media/Files/Report%20Files/2007/Long-Term-Health-Effects-of-Participation-in-Project-SHAD-Shipboard-Hazard-and-Defense/SHAD%20Response%20Letter.pdf (accessed October 7, 2015).

VA (Department of Veterans Affairs). 2002. *VA contacts "Project SHAD" veterans.* http://www.va.gov/opa/pressrel/pressrelease.cfm?id=457 (accessed October 27, 2015).

VA. 2015. *Public health: Agent Orange Registry health exam for veterans.* http://www.publichealth.va.gov/exposures/agentorange/benefits/registry-exam.asp (accessed October 26, 2015).

WHO (World Health Organization). 2015. *International Classification of Diseases (ICD).* http://www.who.int/classifications/icd/en (accessed August 4, 2015).

# Appendix A

# Committee and Consultant Biographies

## COMMITTEE MEMBERS

**David J. Tollerud, M.D., M.P.H.** (*Chair*), is professor and chair of the Department of Environmental and Occupational Health Sciences at the University of Louisville School of Public Health and Information Sciences. He received his M.D. from Mayo Medical School in 1978 and his M.P.H. from the Harvard School of Public Health in 1990. Dr. Tollerud has extensive clinical training, with specialty board certifications in internal medicine, pulmonary and critical care medicine, and environmental and occupational medicine, with a longstanding interest in the health of disadvantaged and underserved populations. Dr. Tollerud's research interests include the effects of environmental pollution on asthma and other health problems, particularly among children and inner-city disadvantaged populations; the influence of cigarette smoke on human health, particularly the immune system; obesity and diabetes research, both the immunological aspects and environmental influences; and hematopoietic stem-cell transplants. An additional area of research interest is strategies to prevent work-related injury and illness. Dr. Tollerud has published more than 90 scientific articles, books, and book chapters; is a member of numerous professional and scientific organizations; and sits on a number of local, national, and international committees dealing with environmental, occupational, and public health issues. In addition to chairing the National Academies of Sciences, Engineering, and Medicine Committee on Shipboard Hazard and Defense II (SHAD II), he served as chair of the Institute of Medicine (IOM) Committee on Air Force Health Study (Ranch Hand) Data and Biospecimens Available for Research. He previously chaired the IOM Committee on the Long-Term Health Consequences of Exposure to Burn Pits in Iraq and Afghanistan; and he has served in various capacities on almost a dozen IOM and National Research Council (NRC) committees, studies, and boards.

**Joseph A. Boscarino, Ph.D., M.P.H.,** is a senior epidemiologist and behavioral scientist at the Geisinger Center for Health Research. Over the past 35 years, he has directed hundreds of studies related to HIV disease, chronic hepatitis, cardiovascular disease, cancer, rheumatoid arthritis, patient satisfaction, addictions, and other topics conducted in the contract research, organizational, and academic settings. His current funded research at Geisinger Clinic includes assessing the outcomes for chronic hepatitis B and C infections, the onset and course of primary biliary cirrhosis, and the use of naloxone in prevention of opioid overdose mortality. Dr. Boscarino is presently the site principal investigator (PI) for the Chronic Hepatitis Cohort Study (CHeCS), funded by the Centers for Disease Control and Prevention Foundation, and was the site PI for the Stevens–Johnson Syndrome Study (funded by the Food and Drug Administration) and a colorectal cancer study (funded by the National Cancer Institute). Currently, he is also evaluating the impact of Hurricane Sandy and a collaborative mental health intervention for Meridian Health in New Jersey, funded by the New Jersey Department of Health. Dr. Boscarino has been funded by the National Institutes of Health (NIH) to study the health impact of the World Trade Center Disaster in New York City and to develop the next generation of posttraumatic stress disorder (PTSD) prediction tools for use in clinical practice (i.e., New York PTSD Risk Score). Before joining Geisinger, he was a senior scientist with the New York Academy of Medicine in New York City and a senior director with Merck-Medco in Franklin Lakes, New Jersey. Dr. Boscarino currently holds adjunct appointments at Mount Sinai School of Medicine (Associate Professor, Medicine and Pediatrics) and at Temple University School of Medicine (Professor, Psychiatry). In 2009, he was elected to Fellow Status by the American Psychological Association (APA) and in 2010 received a Lifetime Achievement Award from the International Society for Traumatic Stress Studies (ISTSS) for his research. Dr. Boscarino is currently a member of the APA, ISTSS, the Society of Biological Psychiatry, and the American College of Epidemiology. Dr. Boscarino is a Vietnam combat veteran; he served in the U.S. Army from August 1964 to December 1966, including 13 months as a combat artilleryman assigned to the II Corps Theater of Operations.

**Linda A. McCauley, R.N., Ph.D.,** is professor and dean of the Nell Hodgson Woodruff School of Nursing at Emory University. A nurse epidemiologist who conducts occupational and environmental health research, her work focuses primarily on chemical exposures and effects on health, including neurobehavioral function and biomarkers of DNA damage. She has conducted large epidemiological investigations of health effects associated with deployment in the 1991 Gulf War and has published numerous papers on exposure assessment and symptoms of veterans of that conflict, including those of troops exposed to chemical warfare agents detonated at the Khamisyah site. Dr. McCauley also led a large research program on organophosphate pesticide exposures in workers and their children in the agricultural communities in the northwest United States. She currently continues her research program on pesticide exposures in agricultural and urban populations. A major focus of her research includes partnering with communities and broad stakeholder involvement in both research participation and dissemination of research findings. Dr. McCauley is particularly known for her community-based participatory research methods with vulnerable populations at risk for environmental exposures. Among the other IOM/NRC committees she served on are the Committee for Review of the Health Effects in Vietnam Veterans of Exposure to Herbicides (Eighth) Biennial Update; the Post-Vietnam Dioxin Exposure in Agent Orange–Contaminated C-123 Aircraft, and the Roundtable on Environmental Health Sciences, Research, and Medicine. She was elected to membership in the National Academy of Medicine in 2008 (at the time called the IOM) and currently serves on the Academies Board on Population Health and Public Health Practice.

**Thomas E. McKone, Ph.D.,** is a senior staff scientist and deputy division director at the Lawrence Berkeley National Laboratory and a professor of environmental health sciences at University of California, Berkeley, School of Public Health. Dr. McKone is a fellow of the Society for Risk Analysis, a former president of the International Society of Exposure Analysis, and a member of the Organizing Committee for the International Life-Cycle Initiative, which is a joint effort of the United Nations Environment Programme and the Society for Environmental Toxicology and Chemistry. His research interests include the use of multimedia compartment models in health-risk assessments, chemical transport and transformation in the environment, and measuring and modeling the biophysics of contaminant transport from the environment into the microenvironments with which humans have contact and across the human–environment exchange boundaries—skin, lungs, and gut. One of Dr. McKone's most recognized achievements was his development of the CalTOX risk-assessment framework for the California Environmental Protection Agency (CalEPA). In 2007, he was appointed by the governor to the Scientific Guidance Panel of the California Environmental Contaminant Biomonitoring Program and continues to serve on this panel. Dr. McKone also served on National Institute for Environmental Health Sciences National Advisory Environmental Health Sciences Council. He is currently a member of the Academies Board on Environmental Studies and Toxicology and has been a member of several NRC committees, including the Committee on Environmental Decision Making: Principles and Criteria for Models, the Committee on Improving Risk Analysis Approaches Used by the U.S. EPA, the Committee on Human Health Reassessment of TCDD and Related Compounds, and the Subcommittee on Zinc Cadmium Sulfide. He served as PI for the NRC study on Strategies to Protect the Health of Deployed U.S. Forces: Detecting, Characterizing, and Documenting Exposures.

**Kenneth R. Still, Ph.D.,** is a retired U.S. Navy captain (O-6) in the Medical Service Corps. Dr. Still completed his Navy career as the senior director of the Navy Occupational Health and Safety Program for the commander of the U.S. Pacific Fleet, Pearl Harbor, Hawaii. Previously, he was the Officer-in-Charge of the Navy's Toxicology Research Laboratory and Program, located in Dayton, Ohio. Dr. Still retired from the U.S. Navy in November 2005 and is currently the scientific director and senior toxicology and industrial hygiene consultant for Occupational Toxicology Associates, Inc., Lake Oswego, Oregon. He chaired an independent toxicology panel for an international corporation addressing risk and exposure assessment for more than 1,700 chemicals and has provided consulting services for several Department of Defense programs, including the Breast Cancer Research Program under the aegis of the Congressionally Directed Medical Research Program. He currently holds an adjunct professorship at Portland State University, School of Community Health, where he teaches graduate and undergraduate courses in environmental health, and is active in the Oregon Masters of Public Health Program. Dr. Still's research has addressed the areas of neurobehavioral, reproductive, inhalation/respiratory, biochemical, and occupational toxicology. He received Vice President Al Gore's Hammer Award for Reinventing Government for work on the EPA Acute Exposure Guidelines. Dr. Still has more than 250 publications in the areas of his research. He holds certifications in the comprehensive practice of industrial hygiene, toxicology, safety, hazardous materials management, and several environmental arenas including environmental auditing and management. He is a fellow of the Academy of Toxicological Sciences and of the American Industrial Hygiene Association. Dr. Still is currently serving on the Academies Committee on Toxicology, the Acute Exposure Guidelines Committee, and the Spacecraft Exposure Guidelines

Committee. He received an M.B.A. in financial management from Chaminade University of Honolulu, an M.S. in physiological ecology from Portland State University, and his Ph.D. in physiological ecology from Oklahoma State University. Dr. Still previously served on the IOM Committee for Presumptive Disability Decision Making Process and the Committee on Blue Water Navy Vietnam Veterans and Agent Orange Exposure.

**Beth A. Virnig, Ph.D., M.P.H.,** is a professor and senior associate dean for academic affairs and research at the University of Minnesota (UMN) School of Public Health. She has a doctorate in epidemiology and is an expert in the use of Medicare and other administrative data for studying health care use and outcomes. She is principal investigator of the UMN DEcIDE comparative effectiveness center and is an investigator with the Research Data Assistance Center and the Women's Health Initiative. Her work focuses on clinical research, including late effects of care, access to care, and the role of health care on disease outcomes. She is a member of the Delta Omega Public Health Honor Society.

**Yiliang Zhu, Ph.D.,** is a professor in the Department of Epidemiology and Biostatistics of the College of Public Health at the University of South Florida where he directs the college's Center for Collaborative Research and the Biostatistics Ph.D. program. He is also a professor of internal medicine in the Morsani College of Medicine at the University of South Florida. From 2013 to 2015 he was a research fellow with the EPA as a Science and Technology Policy Fellow of the American Association for Advancement of Science. Prior to that he was a 2012-2013 Fulbright Fellow in China where he launched the Loess Health Project, a 15-year cohort study of rural health and policy in northwestern China. His current research is focused on health risk assessment, including integrative system modeling based on adverse outcome pathways; exposure to indoor health hazards; evaluation of health care policies, systems, and health outcomes; and biostatistical methods for spatiotemporal data. Dr. Zhu has served as a member of a number of Academies committees, including those on the EPA's assessment of dioxin and related compounds, tetrachloroethylene, and formaldehyde, and the Committees on Science for the Future of EPA and on the EPA's IRIS Process Review. He was also a member of the Department of Health and Human Services' Advisory Committee of Organ Transplantation.

## CONSULTANTS

**Daniel H. Freeman, Jr., Ph.D.,** is a Professor Emeritus of Preventive Medicine and Community Health (Biostatistics) and former director of the Office of Biostatistics at the University of Texas Medical Branch at Galveston. He has a doctorate in biostatistics from the University of North Carolina at Chapel Hill. He has served on the faculty at Yale University School of Public Health, Dartmouth Medical School, and the University of Puerto Rico School of Public Health. He has published more than 200 scientific papers and one monograph, *Applied Categorical Data Analysis.*

**Cynthia C. Johnson** is a medical records and health information technician at the Virginia Department of Health Statistics in Richmond. She is a certified medical classification specialist/nosologist with training from the National Center for Health Statistics in using International Classification of Disease mortality coding. She has considerable experience in interpreting, coding, and classifying medical mortality, multiple cause of death, and underlying cause of death using procedures governed by the National Center for Health Statistics.

**Alfred K. Mbah, Ph.D.,** is a biostatistician, with extensive experience in data analysis applied to health sciences. He is currently an assistant professor in the Department of Epidemiology and Biostatistics in the College of Public Health at the University of South Florida. Dr. Mbah has co-authored numerous peer-reviewed articles. He has served as the lead statistician on multiple studies that examine health disparities and has taught numerous courses in various areas of statistics for more than 7 years.

**James E. Quinn, M.S.,** is a retired U.S. Navy Commander (Surface Warfare Specialist and Marine Transportation Subspecialist). He served in small combatants (destroyer escorts, destroyers, and guided missile destroyers) in weapons, operations, and executive billets. Assignments ashore included operations instructor at the U.S. Naval Academy, Senior Riverine Warfare advisor to the South Vietnamese Navy, and fleet operations assignments with the Military Sealift Command. He graduated from the U.S. Naval War College (Command and Staff) and earned his M.S. in management from the U.S. Naval Postgraduate School. Following retirement from the Navy, he served for 20 years as an operations specialist in a number of contracts with the Departments of Defense and Energy.

# Appendix B

# Agendas for Information-Gathering Meetings

**MEETING 1**
Thursday, January 19, 2012
Keck Center of the National Academies
Washington, DC

**12:45 p.m.** **Introductory Remarks**
*David J. Tollerud, M.D., M.P.H.*
*Chair, Committee on Shipboard Hazard and Defense II*

Introductions by committee members and meeting attendees

**1:00 p.m.** **Study Context and Goals, Congressional Perspective**
*Timothy Daly*
*Legislative Director*
*Office of Congressman Mike Thompson*

Questions and discussion with the committee

**1:30 p.m.** **Study Context and Goals, Sponsor Perspective**
*Wendi Dick, M.D., M.P.H., M.C.R.P.*
*Co-Director, Environmental Health Program, Post-Deployment Health Strategic Healthcare Group, Office of Public Health*
*Veterans Health Administration*

Questions and discussion with the committee

**2:00 p.m.** **The Why, How, and What We Know About SHAD Testing**
*Michael E. Kilpatrick, M.D.*
*Deputy Director, Force Health Protection and Readiness Programs*
*Military Health System, Department of Defense*

Questions and discussion with the committee

**2:45 p.m.** **Methods and Findings from First Institute of Medicine SHAD Study**
*Institute of Medicine Staff*

**3:15 p.m. Break**

**3:30 p.m. Veterans' Perspectives on SHAD Testing**

*Jack Alderson, U.S. Navy Reserve (Ret.)*
*Ferndale, California*

*Norman LaChapelle, M.S.P.H.*
*Commander, Military Sealift Command, U.S. Navy (Ret.)*
*(by phone)*

Questions and discussion with the committee

**4:15 p.m. Additional SHAD Veterans' Experiences**

*Ivian "I.C." Smith*
*Laneview, Virginia*

*George James Brocklebank (by phone)*
*Tuscaloosa, Alabama*

*Terry G. Hansen (by phone)*
*St. George, Utah*

*Alexander Bass (by phone)*
*Jaffrey, New Hampshire*

*Daniel Finn (by phone) [did not speak]*
*Carollton, Alabama*

*Thomas E. Gwise, Ed.D. (by phone)*
*Merritt Island, Florida*

*Dale Hunter (by phone)*
*Hertford, North Carolina*

**5:20 p.m. Opportunity for Additional Public Comment**

*Eric Longabardi*
*Producer/Investigative Journalist*
*TeleMedia News Productions*

**5:30 p.m. Opportunity for Comment by Veterans Service Organizations**

*Rick Weidman*
*Vietnam Veterans of America*

**5:45 p.m. Adjourn Open Session**

**MEETING 2**
Thursday, February 23, 2012
Hyatt Regency
Sacramento, CA

**9:00 a.m.** **Introductory Remarks**
*David J. Tollerud, M.D., M.P.H.*
*Chair, Committee on Shipboard Hazard and Defense II*

Introductions by committee members and meeting attendees

**9:15 a.m.** **Study Context and Goals, Congressional Perspective**
*Congressman Mike Thompson*
*[Remarks conveyed by phone by Mr. Tim Daly, Legislative Director]*

Questions and discussion with the committee

**10:00 a.m.** **Break**

**10:15 a.m.** **Panel Discussions: Project SHAD Experiences**

Panel I: Project SHAD Technical Staff

*Jack Alderson, LCDR USNR (Ret.)*
*Officer in Charge, Project SHAD Technical Staff Tug Division*

*Jack Barry*
*Deseret Test Center*
*Civilian, Test and Plans Officer (Ret.)*

*William D. Bridge, LCDR USN (Ret.)*
*1st Officer in Charge, Project SHAD Technical Staff*

*Robert Kinsella, HMC, USN (Ret.) (phone)*
*Project SHAD Technical Staff Logistic Support*

*Norman LaChapelle, M.S.P.H., CMDR, USN (Ret.)*
*Military Sealift Command*

*Ed McQueen*
*Officer in Charge, LT 2081*

Questions and discussion with committee

**12:00 p.m.** **Break for Lunch**

**1:00 p.m.** **SHAD and Human Test Subjects: Exposure, Dissemination, Dosage, and Penetration**

*Eric Longabardi*
*Producer/Investigative Journalist*
*TeleMedia News Productions*

Questions and discussion with committee

**1:30 p.m.** **Panel Discussions: Project SHAD Experiences (Continued)**

Panel II: Veterans with SHAD Test Experiences

*George Arnold*
*Veteran from the USS* Navarro *[Autumn Gold]*
*Hay Fork, California*

*Robert Bates (by phone)*
*Veteran from the USS* Navarro *[Autumn Gold]*
*Vancouver, Washington*

*John Ekman*
*Veteran from the USS* Power *[Copper Head]*

*John Goricki (by phone)*
*Veteran from the USS* Power *[Copper Head]*
*Ft. Meyers, Florida*

Questions and discussion with committee

**3:15 p.m.** **Break**

**3:30 p.m.** **Panel Discussions: Project SHAD Experiences (Continued)**

Panel III: Veterans Involved in DTC Test 69-10

*Ray Batiato (by phone)*
*Veteran from the USS* Fort Snelling

*Mike Coneys (by phone)*
*Veteran from the USS* Fort Snelling

*Daniel Finn (by phone)*
*Veteran from the USS* Fort Snelling
*Carollton, Alabama*

*Ozzie Kariman (by phone) CANCELLED*
*Veteran of 1st Battalion, 8th Marines, B Company*
*Lockport, New York*

*Wayne Kiekenbush (by phone)*
*Veteran from the USS* Fort Snelling

*Adrian Szarowicz Jr. (by phone) CANCELLED*
*Veteran from the USS* Fort Snelling

Questions and discussion with committee

**4:30 p.m.** **Additional Aspects of SHAD Veterans' Experiences**
*Robert Rinehart*

**5:00 p.m.** **Adjourn Open Session**

# Appendix C

## Review of Literature on Known Project SHAD Agents, Simulants, Tracers, and Decontaminants

At the committee's request, the Institute of Medicine (IOM) research librarian carried out targeted literature searches on the following agents, simulants, tracers, and decontaminants[1]:

1. *Bacillus globigii* (BG)
2. Betapropiolactone (beta-propiolactone; BPL)
3. Calcium hypochlorite
4. Calcofluor
5. *Coxiella burnetii* (CB, Q fever)
6. Diethylphthalate (DEP)
7. *Escherichia coli* (*E.coli*; EC)
8. Methyl acetoacetate (MAA)
9. *Pasteurella tularensis* (*Francisella tularensis*)
10. Phenol
11. Sarin
12. *Serratia marcescens* (SM)
13. Staphylococcal enterotoxin type B (SEB)
14. Sulfur dioxide
15. Trioctyl phosphate (TOF)
16. Uranine
17. VX nerve agent (VX)
18. Zinc cadmium sulfide

These searches were conducted to determine whether new information was available to update the reviews of these materials that had been prepared in 2004 for the SHAD I study (IOM, 2007b).[2] The searches were designed to identify peer-reviewed literature published

---

[1] The SHAD I (IOM, 2007b) review included bis-hydrogen phosphite and phosphorus-32, but these substances were not included in the updated review of literature for this study. These tracers were disseminated with VX over a barge in the Flower Drum II test. No personnel have been identified as participants in this test.

[2] The SHAD I report is available for free download at http://iom.nationalacademies.org/Reports/2007/Long-Term-Health-Effects-of-Participation-in-Project-SHAD-Shipboard-Hazard-and-Defense.aspx (accessed December 7,

between January 2001 and January 2012 on studies in vitro, in animals, or in humans that evaluated the safety or potential long-term health effects of exposure to the substances. The committee did not examine papers reporting use of a given substance in laboratory procedures without evaluation of health effects, papers in which the substance was not the focus of the study, or papers that did not address potential long-term effects of exposure. The databases searched were Medline, Toxline, Embase, Science Citation Index within the Web of Science, Chemical Carcinogenesis Research Information System (CCRIS), Hazardous Substances Data Bank (HSDB), and Integrated Risk Information System (IRIS). The searches used the substance name, synonyms, and the Chemical Abstracts Service (CAS) registry number, as appropriate.

The descriptions that follow summarize findings from background papers prepared by the Center for Research Information (CRI) for the SHAD I study (IOM, 2007b). They also reflect new findings or additional information drawn from the supplemental literature searches. The committee sought to generate hypotheses that it could use to provide some focus for a portion of its analysis. In these descriptions, the committee notes instances where the available literature provides at least some evidence that an exposure *might* be associated with an increased risk of certain long-term health effects. The committee is using "long-term" to mean persisting, recurring, or appearing several years or more after exposure. The committee's identification of a health effect means that it was judged to warrant investigation as an a priori hypothesis to be tested; it does not constitute an assertion by the committee that the evidence is conclusive that the health effect could result from the relatively short-term exposures to the substance that occurred in SHAD tests.

***Bacillus globigii* (*B. globigii* or BG)** [biological simulant]

*B. globigii* is a Gram-positive spore-forming bacterium commonly found in dust, soil, and water and frequently used as a tracer and simulant for spore-forming bacteria such as Bacillus anthracis (e.g., Clark Burton et al., 2005; Duncan et al., 2009) or other bacterial spores (Probst et al., 2010). It has also been called *B. subtilis var niger* and *B. lichenformis*, but it is now referred to as *B. atrophaeus*. BG was used as a simulant in SHAD testing.

The literature search for BG/*B. atrophaeus* did not identify new information on potential long-term health effects from BG exposure or reports of long-term persistence or delayed manifestations of infection. As a result, the committee did not find it necessary to augment the information reported for the SHAD I study (IOM, 2007b) on the potential pathogenicity of BG. As noted in that report, BG was previously considered to be a largely harmless agent, but it is now recognized as a human pathogen. Infection is most often associated with invasive trauma or a weakened health state. Reported effects include ocular infections, bacteremia, sepsis/septicemia, ventriculitis, and peritonitis. Gastrointestinal (GI) effects may occur with consumption of contaminated food. Although these reported short-term health effects can be serious, there are no reports to indicate persistent health consequences once short-term effects have resolved (CRI, 2004a).

---

2015). A set of commissioned papers that reviewed the health-effects literature on these substances were prepared by the Center for Research Information for the first IOM SHAD study and are available at this same website. These commissioned papers are cited in this report as (CRI, 2004[x]).

Studies of *B. globigii*, *B. subtilis* var *niger*, *B. lichenformis*, and *B. atrophaeus* provided no evidence for identifying specific long-term health effects that might be associated with exposure during SHAD testing.

**Betapropiolactone (BPL)** [decontaminant]

BPL is a colorless liquid with a pungent odor that was used in Project SHAD as a decontaminant. Its short-term effects are irritation of the skin, eyes, and respiratory and digestive systems. Dermal exposure can cause blisters and burns, and animal testing has indicated that ocular administration results in pain and corneal opacity. Animal testing has also shown an association between respiratory exposure and inflammation of the respiratory tract.

Human testing to evaluate BPL as an anti-hepatitis disinfectant for plasma transfusion took place at the Henry Ford Hospital in the 1950s and 1960s (Kelly et al., 1957, and LoGrippo, 1964, as cited in CRI, 2004f). No chronic toxic effects were reported in the 995 recipients of treated plasma who were followed for periods ranging from 6 months to 5 years; however, related animal experiments demonstrated cumulative toxicity manifested in weight loss and necrosis of the liver and kidney tubules (Kelly et al., 1957, and LoGrippo, 1964, as cited in CRI, 2004f).

BPL is categorized as a possible human carcinogen (Group 2B) by the International Agency for Research on Cancer (IARC, 1999a), and it is a confirmed animal carcinogen, frequently used in animal experiments to induce cancer (CRI, 2004f). The National Toxicology Program (NTP) categorizes BPL as "reasonably anticipated to be a human carcinogen," based on evidence of carcinogenicity from studies in animals (NTP, 2011, p. 366). Tumor sites reported in experimental animal studies vary with the route of exposure. Oral exposure caused cancer of the stomach, dermal exposure caused benign and malignant skin tumors, and subcutaneous injection caused cancer at the injection site. Lymphoma and liver tumors were also observed following injection. Intrarectal exposure caused benign colon tumors, and inhalation exposure caused cancer of the nasal cavity. The NTP review reported that no epidemiological studies were identified that evaluated the association between exposure to BPL and risk of cancer in humans (NTP, 2011).

The committee's literature search for publications since 2001 did not identify new information on potential long-term health effects from BPL exposure beyond those noted in the review for the previous SHAD report (CRI, 2004f).

Because betapropiolactone is considered a possible human carcinogen, the committee tested the hypothesis that exposure is associated with an increased risk among SHAD test participants for the following conditions:

- Any cancers

**Calcium Hypochlorite** [decontaminant]

Calcium hypochlorite is a yellowish-white solid with formula $Ca(ClO)_2$ and CAS number 7778-54-3. It smells strongly of chlorine. It is an ingredient in bleaching powder, and it is used in household cleaners and disinfectants, drinking and wastewater purification systems, and disinfection systems for swimming pools (ATSDR, 2011). It was reported to have been used as a decontaminant in at least two tests carried out as part of Project SHAD.

Calcium hypochlorite was not among the substances for which a literature review was carried out for the first IOM study on the potential long-term health effects from participation in Project SHAD. The literature search for the SHAD II study found limited information available from sources such as the Agency for Toxic Substances and Disease Registry (ATSDR), International Agency for Research on Cancer (IARC), and HSDB. Calcium hypochlorite can be an irritant to the eyes, skin, respiratory tract, and GI tract. At high concentrations it can cause severe damage to these tissues or even death. Dermal exposure to $Ca(ClO)_2$ at high concentrations can cause pain, inflammation, and blisters. Exposure of the eyes can result in effects that range from mild irritation to severe injury, depending on the exposure concentration (ATSDR, 2011). Exposure to chlorine gas released from concentrated calcium hypochlorite solutions can lead to coughing, nasal irritation, and sore throat. Little evidence is available regarding the carcinogenicity of hypochlorite salts in animals, and no data on carcinogenicity were available from human studies. As a result, IARC (1997) determined that calcium hypochlorite is not classifiable regarding its carcinogenicity.

Available studies of calcium hypochlorite provided no evidence for identifying specific long-term health effects that might be associated with exposure during SHAD testing.

**Calcofluor** [tracer]

Calcofluor is a fluorescent whitening agent used to brighten items such as paper and textiles. It is also used as a laboratory stain and as a fluorescent tracer in the environment. It was used as a tracer in the SHAD tests designated Half Note and Test 69-32.

The IOM search for references relevant to potential long-term human health effects from exposure to calcofluor did not identify relevant journal articles published since the literature review carried out for the first SHAD study. That review found that the toxicity of calcofluor is low, based on oral and dermal toxicity studies in fish, mammals, and humans (CRI, 2004g). It has not been found to be carcinogenic or mutagenic to humans.

Studies of calcofluor provided no evidence for identifying specific long-term health effects that might be associated with exposure during SHAD testing.

***Coxiella burnetii* (*C. burnetii* or CB)** [active biological agent]

*C. burnetii* is a bacterium that is the causative agent of Q fever. It was investigated as a potential biological warfare agent during SHAD testing in the 1960s. Its primary natural reservoirs are animals such as cattle, sheep, and goats. Transmission from these animals to humans most frequently occurs through inhalation of aerosolized bacteria shed by animals (CDC, 2011, 2012). The bacterium has an extracellular form that is metabolically inactive, can be transmitted through air and dust, and remains infectious for several weeks in natural environments (CRI, 2004b). Aerosolized *C. burnetii* was used as part of Project SHAD in the test called Shady Grove.

Infection with *C. burnetii* can cause various acute and chronic health effects. However, only about 40 percent of people infected with it report clinical symptoms (CRI, 2004b). According to the Centers for Disease Control and Prevention (CDC), roughly 3 percent of the healthy U.S. population and 10-20 percent of persons in high-risk occupations (veterinarians, farmers, etc.) have antibodies to *C. burnetii* (CDC, 2012).

The acute form of Q fever typically arises 10-17 days after exposure, with common modes of presentation including pneumonia, hepatitis, or an influenza-like febrile illness (IOM, 2007a). Long-term effects from infection with *C. burnetii* have been observed. Neurologic deficits sometimes develop during the acute phase of the illness and can continue over the long term. In addition, the scientific literature links five chronic syndromes with *C. burnetii* infection: endocarditis, vascular infection, chronic hepatitis, osteomyelitis, and a post-Q fever fatigue syndrome (IOM, 2007a). Among these conditions, endocarditis and vascular infection appear to be the most common (Raoult et al., 2000). Of note, acute Q fever is not a necessary precursor for Q fever endocarditis. In a large case series in France only one-third of Q fever endocarditis patients reported potential Q fever in the year before the start of endocarditis symptoms (Raoult et al., 2000). Q fever endocarditis is most common in those with abnormal or prosthetic cardiac valves or underlying cardiac valvular lesions (IOM, 2007a).

The SHAD II committee's examination of the relevant recent literature reinforced the association of *C. burnetii* infection with endocarditis and vascular infection (e.g., Alshukairi et al., 2006; Angelakis and Raoult, 2010). Recent Q fever outbreaks in the Netherlands (Kampschreur et al., 2012) and increasing awareness of the disease elsewhere (Bacci et al., 2012) are providing more information about the natural history and prevalence of the disease. However, long-term effects from *C. burnetii* infection are difficult to study because infection is at times asymptomatic and results of serological testing to identify past infections can vary across reference laboratories using the same immunological test (Healy et al., 2011). Active research on the natural history of *C. burnetii* infection and potential chronic effects of infection is ongoing (Hartzell et al., 2008; Raoult et al., 2005; van der Hoek et al., 2012).

Based on the evidence available regarding potential long-term health effects associated with exposure to *C. burnetii*, the committee tested the hypotheses that participation in SHAD tests that used *C. burnetii* may be associated with increased risk for the following conditions:

- Endocarditis
- Vascular infection
- Chronic hepatitis
- Osteomyelitis
- Post Q-fever fatigue syndrome

**Diethylphthalate (DEP)** [chemical simulant]

DEP is a liquid chemical widely used in industrial and consumer products, including automobile parts, toothbrushes, tools, food packaging, aspirin, insecticides, and cosmetics (CRI, 2004h). It is frequently used to make plastics more flexible (e.g., medical tubing), and in this role is known as a "plasticizer." It was used in Project SHAD as a simulant for VX nerve agent.

Because of wide human exposure to this compound, many studies have been carried out to evaluate its toxicity. Dermal sensitization to DEP has been described but seems to be rare (WHO, 2003). Other than producing irritation of mucous membranes and the lungs and a general anesthetic effect at high doses (CRI, 2004h), it has shown very low toxicity.

Studies in animals of the potential for low doses of phthalates such as DEP to influence immune and allergic responses have not provided consistent answers (Kimber and Dearman, 2010). Recent concerns about the potential for phthalates to disrupt endocrine signaling have led to additional studies evaluating the potential for altered reproductive effects. However, in a study of the comparative toxicology of nine phthalate diesters (including DEP) and five monoesters administered to male rats at high doses, DEP showed only few and subtle effects compared to the other compounds (Kwack et al., 2009). Exposure to DEP in utero did not alter sexual differentiation in male rat pups (Gray et al., 2000). However, a study in which male Wistar rats were fed DEP dissolved in the diet daily for 5 months showed dose-dependent changes in liver histology (Pereira et al., 2006) and Wistar rats continuously exposed to DEP through diet over three generations showed fatty degeneration of the liver, particularly in the third (F2) generation (Pereira et al., 2007). DEP is not among phthalates that have been banned from cosmetics or children's toys by the United States or the European Union (EurActiv, 2004).

Studies of DEP provided no evidence for identifying specific long-term health effects that might be associated with exposure during SHAD testing.

***Escherichia coli* (*E. coli* or EC)** [biological simulant]

*E. coli* is a Gram-negative bacterium that belongs to the Enterobacteriacae family. Large numbers of strains of *E. coli* are known to exist. Many strains are harmless, including ones that commonly inhabit the human intestines (enteric bacteria), and *E. coli* is widely used in laboratories for research. However, certain strains can be significantly pathogenic. *E. coli* was used in Project SHAD as a simulant to study the decay of biological agents in a marine or shipboard environment. Records available to the committee did not specify the strain of *E. coli* used in the SHAD tests, but its use as a simulant suggests avoidance of any strains known to be pathogenic.

Oral exposure to pathogenic strains of *E. coli* can cause diarrhea and nausea, which typically resolve in 1-2 days. *E. coli* is a common source of hospital-acquired infection, as well as a frequent cause of urinary tract and blood infections. Some forms of pathogenic *E. coli* can cause severe and even fatal illness.

The literature search seeking new references since the CRI's 2004 review found several articles of note on health effects of infection with pathogenic forms of *E. coli*. Berger et al. (2010) found risk factors for *E. coli* bacteremia to include vascular catheters, malignancy, and cytoreductive or immunosuppressive therapy. In another study, risk factors for recurrent *E. coli* infections of the bloodstream included being male, the presence of hematologic malignancy, and inadequate antibiotic treatment (Sanz-Garcia et al., 2009). Smith and Bayles (2007) noted that *E.coli* is among several foodborne pathogens commonly associated with postinfectious irritable bowel syndrome. A considerable literature surrounds potential sequelae from infection by the *E. coli* O157:H7 strain. The highly pathogenic *E. coli* O157:H7 was not recognized until the 1980s and is not likely to be relevant to potential effects from Project SHAD exposures.

The use of *E. coli* in SHAD tests as a simulant would seem to suggest that the intention was to select a nonpathogenic strain for this purpose. However, because the specific strain used is not known, the committee considered evidence regarding potential long-term health effects associated with exposure to certain pathogenic strains of *E. coli.* Based on that evidence, the committee tested the hypotheses that participation in SHAD tests that used *E. coli* may be associated with increased risk for the following condition:

- Irritable bowel syndrome

**Methyl Acetoacetate (MAA)** [chemical simulant]

MAA is a colorless liquid frequently used in the fragrance industry. The general population may be exposed through breathing wood smoke (HSDB citing NIOSH, 1983). It was used in Project SHAD as a simulant for the nerve agent sarin.

Methyl acetoacetate is considered to be a mild irritant: exposure may cause swelling, redness, or pain, particularly at mucous membranes (CRI, 2004i), and may cause corrosive effects to the eye. It is not considered to be mutagenic nor has it shown reproductive or developmental effects in the rat (CRI, 2004i; HSDB, 2005). However, studies of the toxicity of MAA are limited. The literature search seeking new reports since the review for the first IOM SHAD study identified only HSDB (2005) information and a summary of mutagenicity studies in CCRIS (2010). All but one of the mutagenicity studies were negative. The positive results in the one study are thought to be an artifact of problems with the pH of the test system (CRI, 2004i).

Studies of MAA provided no evidence for identifying specific long-term health effects that might be associated with exposure during SHAD testing.

***Pasteurella tularensis* (*Francisella tularensis*)** [active biological agent]

*Pasteurella tularensis*, which has been renamed *Francisella tularensis*, is a Gram-negative coccobacillus that is the causative agent for the disease tularemia. It is carried by animals, and its transmission to humans is associated with being in contact with animals or with tick bites. It is also considered to be a possible bioterror agent because of its ability to cause debilitating or fatal illness. Aerosolized *F. tularensis* was used as part of Project SHAD in the test called Shady Grove.

Infection with *F. tularensis* typically results in fever, with additional symptoms such as chills, headaches, weight loss, emesis, diarrhea, muscle aches, joint pain, cough, hepatitis, and jaundice. Local enlargement of the lymph glands, skin eruptions, and ulcerations often occur at the site of initial inoculation. The more common manifestations are in skin, lymph, lungs, and liver. Sometimes patients experience atypical signs and effects such as neuropathies, meningeal involvement, and pericarditis. The typical course of infection is 1 month of fever, 1 month of weakness, and 6 weeks of gradual but complete recovery (CRI, 2004c). However, exposure to aerosolized *F. tularensis* can lead within days or weeks to respiratory failure and death if the infection is untreated (Dennis et al., 2012). Several clinical syndromes have been described and include glandular, pneumonic, and typhoidal forms (CIDRAP, 2010).

Tularemia is considered a “strictly acute disease” (CRI, 2004c, p. 2). Although one case report documents recurrences of fever and ulcerations over a decade, there are no reports of symptoms first appearing months or years after initial infection.

The literature search seeking new references since the CRI review (2004c) did not identify additional papers relevant to potential long-term effects from infection with *F. tularensis*.

Studies of *F. tularensis* and tularemia provided no evidence for identifying specific long-term health effects that might be associated with exposure during SHAD testing.

**Phenol** [noted as component in preparation of simulant BG in Half Note test]

Phenol is an organic compound with the chemical formula $C_6H_6O$ and a sweet and tarry odor. It is manufactured in large amounts in the United States. It is used in the manufacture of plastics, in household cleaning products, and in consumer products such as mouthwashes, gargles, throat lozenges, and throat sprays. It is also released into the air in automobile exhaust, cigarette smoke, and smoke from burning wood. Low levels are found in certain smoked and fried foods (ATSDR, 2008). It is used medically as a treatment for spasticity (Cullu et al., 2005; Goktepe et al., 2002; Jarrett et al., 2002; Kolaski et al., 2008; Pinder et al., 2008) and for certain dermatological conditions (Iglesias et al., 2008; Kaminaka et al., 2009a,b). It is also sometimes used as a preservative in vaccines and biologics (Geier et al., 2010). A report on one SHAD test (DTC, 1968) noted that it was added at 1 percent to slurry preparations of BG.

Phenol was not among the substances for which a literature review was carried out for the first IOM study on Project SHAD. The literature search for the current study found an array of publications about health effects of phenol exposure. Most of these reports, such as ATSDR (2008) and HSDB (2003a) summaries, emphasize short-term hazards. Phenol is caustic to tissues, and toxicity can result from oral, dermal, or inhalation exposure. Ingestion of concentrated phenol can cause GI damage and even death. When concentrated phenol is applied to the skin, it can cause burns and other skin damage, as well as liver and kidney toxicity. The National Institute for Occupational Safety and Health (NIOSH, 2011) has assigned a special skin notation for phenol because skin contact can be life-threatening as well as injurious to the skin. Inhalation can result in pulmonary irritation and edema. At high doses dermal absorption can lead to systemic toxicity, including cardiovascular effects, pulmonary depression, and central nervous system effects (NIOSH, 2011). Phenol is considered a weak clastogen (cause of breaks in chromosomes) based on studies in mice (Bruce et al., 2001).

Assessments by IARC (1999b) and Bruce et al. (2001) examined data regarding cancer and other potential long-term endpoints. Phenol has not been shown to be a carcinogen in animals or humans (IARC, 1999b). Information about other potential long-term effects from studies in humans is very limited, but includes reports suggesting the potential for suppression of immune response, altered hematological parameters, and increased liver enzymes in workers (Bruce et al., 2001).

Taken together, the available studies of phenol provided no evidence for identifying specific long-term health effects that might be associated with exposure to phenol during SHAD testing.

**Sarin** [active nerve agent]

Sarin is an organophosphate compound and chemical warfare agent developed by German scientists in the late 1930s. It is a nerve agent that inhibits enzymes known as acetylcholinesterases (AChEs), which are responsible for breaking down the neurotransmitter acetylcholine into choline and acetic acid. With inhibition of the enzymes, the neurotransmitter builds up at nerve synapses to overstimulate nerve receptors. It was a test agent in the SHAD test Flower Drum I.

Health effects from sarin depend on the amount, timing, and route of exposure. Short-term (acute) effects of exposure to sarin at low concentrations include ocular pain, blurred or dimmed vision, miosis (constricted pupils), tearing, runny nose, and sweating. At high concentrations, the effects include convulsions, loss of consciousness, paralysis, and respiratory failure possibly leading to death.

Long-term effects in humans from exposure to sarin have been studied in several populations: those exposed through the terrorist use of sarin in Japan in 1994 and 1995, intentionally exposed military volunteers, accidentally exposed industrial workers, and Gulf War veterans. These studies are reviewed in two IOM reports prepared as part of the Gulf War and Health series (IOM, 2000, 2004). Many methodological challenges accompany epidemiologic studies of exposed populations. Exposure levels are typically uncertain or approximate, and studies have frequently relied on self-report to assess health outcomes. Taking into account the evidence available on the effects of high-dose exposures, the IOM Gulf War and Health committee found "limited/suggestive evidence of an association between exposure to sarin at doses sufficient to cause acute cholinergic signs and symptoms and a variety of subsequent long-term neurological effects" (IOM, 2004, p. 93).

With regard to long-term effects from *low* doses of sarin (exposures "insufficient to cause acute cholinergic signs and symptoms"), the IOM Gulf War and Health committee found "inadequate/insufficient evidence to determine whether an association does or does not exist between exposure" and subsequent long-term adverse neurological health effects (IOM, 2004, p. 96). The review examined evidence on a wide array of general neurological effects (e.g., changes in memory, difficulty in sleeping, cognitive dysfunction) as well as posttraumatic stress disorder. That committee did not believe that it was possible to extrapolate the long-term, low-level effects of organophosphorus (OP) compounds used as insecticides to the case of sarin (IOM, 2004, p. 97).[3]

Since that review, various studies have provided additional data from human studies of long-term effects from sarin exposure. A survey by Kawada et al. (2005) of victims of the Tokyo subway sarin release has observed poorer sleep quality among those in the exposed group compared to a control group. A report by Miyaki et al. (2005) describes decrements in results for certain neurobehavioral tests in a small sample of Tokyo sarin victims 7 years after the sarin exposure. Yamasue et al. (2007) examined the brain morphology of a subset of victims of the

---

[3] Sarin and VX share a mechanism of action with organophosphate compounds used as insecticides: the inhibition of cholinesterases, enzymes that act to break down acetylcholine at nerve synapses. The resulting buildup of acetylcholine leads to some shared symptoms upon exposure to OP insecticides and nerve agents such as sarin and VX. As a result, the potential long-term health effects of low-dose exposure to organophosphate insecticides are of interest.

The IOM committee responsible for *Gulf War and Health, Volume 2: Insecticides and Solvents* (IOM, 2003) reviewed the epidemiologic literature on OP compounds, and found limited/suggestive evidence of associations between chronic exposure to OP insecticides and both non-Hodgkin's lymphoma and adult leukemia. More recently, data from the Agricultural Health Study showed leukemia risk to be elevated in those with highest exposure to fonofos, an organothiophosphate, and identified a significant dose-response trend for lifetime exposure-days and risk of prostate cancer among pesticide applicators with a family history of prostate cancers (Mahajan et al., 2006). Prostate cancer risk was unrelated to fonofos use overall. Mills and Yang (2003) observed an association between increased prostate cancer risk and relatively high levels of several different pesticides, including the organophosphate dichlorvos. A connection between organophosphate pesticides and cancer remains uncertain, and the implications for cancer risk from sarin and VX exposure are also uncertain. As noted, the IOM Committee on Gulf War and Health: Updated Literature Review of Sarin did not believe that it was possible to extrapolate the long-term, low-level effects of OP insecticides to the case of sarin and cyclosarin (IOM, 2004). "Although the OP insecticides and the OP nerve agents are known to share a mechanism of action underlying their acute effects (inhibition of cholinesterase), the mechanism that underlies any potential low-level effects of OP insecticides is less established" (IOM, 2004, p. 97).

1995 subway attack who had been treated in the emergency room for sarin intoxication. Compared to controls, the subjects with sarin exposure had smaller than normal volumes in certain brain regions, correlating with decreased serum cholinesterase levels and the severity of chronic somatic complaints. A report by Yanagisawa et al. (2006) noted the continuation of psychological symptoms after 5 years in some victims of the Matsumoto and Tokyo subway terrorist events.

Experimental studies in animals of long-term effects from sarin exposures have suggested the potential for alterations in muscarinic receptors, suggestive of a potential mechanism through which sarin could cause long-term effects on the nervous system (Henderson et al., 2002; IOM, 2004). Some other changes have been observed in brain histopathology and electroencephalogram (EEG) patterns that persisted for months or up to 1 year. However, these changes did not appear to be associated with behavioral changes or clinically relevant results (IOM, 2004), and it is not clear how to interpret these findings for humans. Experimental studies in animals have not provided evidence of reproductive or developmental toxicity, or of carcinogenicity (CRI, 2004j; IOM, 2004; Munro et al., 1994).

Based on the evidence available regarding potential long-term health effects associated with exposure to sarin, the committee tested the hypotheses that participation in SHAD tests that used sarin may be associated with increased risk for the following conditions:

- Neurological effects
- Psychological symptoms

***Serratia marcescens* (*S. marcescens* or SM)** [biological simulant]

*S. marcescens* is a rod-shaped, Gram-negative bacterium found frequently in soil, water, sewage, foods, and various animals. It is a saprophyte, obtaining nutrients from dead organic material, and is commonly found growing in damp spaces such as bathrooms, where its growth can manifest as a pinkish film. *S. marcescens* was used in Project SHAD to measure the degradation of an aerosolized bacterium as a result of sun exposure in a marine environment. At the time of the SHAD tests it was seen as harmless, but its potential to cause opportunistic infections has since been recognized.

As reviewed by CRI (2004d) for the SHAD I report, *S. marcescens* infection is seen most often as an opportunistic infection in health care settings. It is frequently associated with use of invasive devices or procedures or found in persons with compromised or suppressed immune systems. The infection can result in a variety of health effects involving nearly every physiological system (reviewed in Mahlen, 2011). These effects can include septicemia, urinary tract infections, endocarditis, otitis media, and soft-tissue or skin infections such as necrotizing fasciitis. *S. marcescens* can survive on soft contact lenses and can cause conjunctivitis and infective keratitis. *S. marcescens* strains are frequently resistant to antibiotics. The infections can be lethal.

The new literature search primarily identified reports of cases of *S. marcescens* infection in patients, often with compromised immunity. The conditions reported include skin and other abscesses (Baggish and Nadiminti, 2007; Friedman et al., 2003; Friend et al., 2009; Langrock et al., 2008; Soria et al., 2008; Yoshida et al., 2009), necrotizing fasciitis (Bachmeyer et al., 2004; Liangpunsakul and Pursell, 2001; Wen, 2012), endocarditis (Dokic et al., 2004), granuloma (Yoshihiro et al., 2010), eye infections (Hume and Willcox, 2004; Mah-Sadorra et al., 2005), and central nervous system infections (Huang et al., 2001). The committee did not identify additional evidence of long-term health effects from *S. marcescens* infection that are not connected with an acute or recurring infection.

Studies of *S. marcescens* provided no evidence for identifying specific long-term health effects that might be associated with exposure during the SHAD testing.

**Staphylococcal enterotoxin type B (SEB)** [active biological agent]

SEB is produced by the infectious pathogen *Staphylococcus aureus*. Because of this toxin's ability to cause acute incapacitating illness, it was part of the U.S. biological weapons stockpile. According to DoD (2002), it was used in Project SHAD in the test Speckled Start.

As noted in the literature review for the first SHAD report (CRI, 2004e; IOM, 2007b), SEB can cause adverse health effects through oral, inhalation, and dermal routes of exposure. Oral exposure to SEB can result in symptoms of nausea, vomiting, cramping abdominal pain, and diarrhea. Fever, tachycardia, hypotension, and diffuse abdominal pain are among other possible symptoms. Symptoms from oral exposure typically appear within 1 to 6 hours and resolve within as little as 24 hours. Exposure through inhalation also usually results in symptoms within a few hours, but they last 1 to 2 weeks. High fever is typically followed by myalgia, headache, chills, chest pain, rales, dyspnea, and a nonproductive cough. Nausea and vomiting may also occur. Death is uncommon, although severe and even fatal septic shock is possible as a result of exposure to large doses (CRI, 2004e).

Seemingly independent of its acute effects, SEB acts as a "superantigen" (Fraser, 2011). At minutely low (picomolar) concentrations it strongly activates the immune system (both T-lymphocytes and antigen-presenting cells). SEB exposure can also induce unresponsiveness in memory T-cells and programmed death in cells that initially proliferate. This may be a mechanism through which *S. aureus* evades the immune system (CRI, 2004e).

Long-term effects of SEB exposure may include the start or exacerbation of allergic diseases such as atopic dermatitis, psoriasis vulgaris, vernal keratoconjunctivitis, and atopic keratoconjunctivitis. It has also been associated with the induction of autoimmune diseases such as Graves' disease, rheumatoid arthritis, and multiple sclerosis (CRI, 2004e).

Since the review by CRI, several publications have reiterated or further explored the risk for allergic disease as a potential long-term effect from SEB exposure. For example, J. H. Lee et al. (2005) demonstrated an association between sensitization to Staphylococcal enterotoxin type A (SEA) and SEB and an increased risk for allergic airway disease such as bronchial asthma. Findings of Liu et al. (2006a,b) supported the potential relationship of SEB with TH2 immune responses in sinusitis and with food allergy. Rajagopalan et al. (2006a,b) demonstrated in mice that intranasal and conjunctival exposure to SEB can cause systemic immune activation. A report based on occupational exposures at the U.S. Army Medical Research Institute of Infectious Diseases notes three cases in which ocular exposures to SEB resulted in conjunctivitis and localized swelling (Rusnak et al., 2004). Tomi et al. (2005) found that the severity of atopic dermatitis and psoriasis correlated with enterotoxin production by *S. aureus* strains isolated from the skin of patients.

Based on the evidence available regarding potential long-term health effects associated with exposure to SEB, the committee identified as possible hypotheses that participation in SHAD tests that used SEB may be associated with increased risk for the following conditions that may reflect heightened allergic responses:

- Asthma
- Rheumatoid arthritis
- Graves' disease
- Multiple sclerosis

However, the committee was not able to test this hypothesis because the study population included too few individuals from the test in which SEB was used.

**Sulfur dioxide ($SO_2$)** [chemical simulant]

$SO_2$ is a colorless gas with a pungent odor. It has many industrial uses and is a component of air pollution. It is also used as a biocide and preservative in the agriculture and food industries (IARC, 1992). It was used as a simulant for the nerve gas sarin in Project SHAD.

Typical exposure to $SO_2$ is through inhalation. At levels higher than the odor threshold, exposure can lead to short-term responses of lung irritation, bronchoconstriction, asthma-like symptoms, and respiratory distress. At sufficiently high levels, exposure can lead to permanent impairment of lung function in the form of reactive airways dysfunction syndrome (RADS), chronic obstructive pulmonary disease (COPD), or enhanced sensitivity in asthmatics (CRI, 2004k). $SO_2$ has also been linked to damage to developing fetuses and the reproductive system, and, with long-term exposure, to low birth weights and in adults to cerebrovascular and heart disease, pulmonary disorders, and increased morbidity and mortality (CRI, 2004k).

Research in cell systems and animals has indicated that $SO_2$ exposure can decrease levels of antioxidant enzymes, cause chromosome breakage, and be mutagenic or comutagenic (CRI, 2004k). The most recent assessment of sulfur dioxide by IARC (1992) found inadequate evidence to determine its carcinogenicity in humans and limited evidence for its carcinogenicity in animals.

The literature search seeking new reports since the 2004 CRI review found continued active research into the health effects of exposure to $SO_2$. Many studies have been done in cell systems or animals. Studies in cultured human bronchial epithelial cells (Li and Meng, 2007, Li et al., 2007a) and male Wistar rats (Li et al., 2007b, 2008) suggest that $SO_2$ increases the expression of certain genes related to asthma, which might be a mechanism through which $SO_2$ aggravates asthma. A series of studies in mice by the same group indicates that $SO_2$ can enter lungs and other organs, such as the heart (Meng et al., 2005), and cause oxidative damage (Meng et al., 2003) and damage to DNA (Meng et al., 2004, 2005). These researchers also found $SO_2$ inhalation to lead to chromosomal aberrations in bone marrow cells (Meng and Zhang, 2002). In contrast, the results of a study by Ziemann et al. (2009) indicated an absence of mutagenicity in a bone marrow micronucleus test with NMRI mice. Studies in rats by Sang et al. (2009, 2010, 2011) have explored the potential mechanisms of neurotoxicity of $SO_2$, finding a likely role for free radicals generated by $SO_2$ metabolism. Zhang et al. (2006a,b) found indications of oxidative stress in the testes of adult male rats exposed to 15 parts per million of $SO_2$ in air for 4 hours per day.

Studies of health effects in humans from exposures to $SO_2$ include observing an increase in the incidence of asthma in workers who experienced repeated peak exposures to $SO_2$ during work at sulfite pulp mills (Andersson et al., 2006). In addition, higher estimated mean exposure to outdoor $SO_2$ was associated with greater lifetime prevalence of asthma diagnosed by a doctor in a study of Czech and Polish school children (Pikhart et al., 2001). A small study of exposure to $SO_2$ over a season of apricot sulfurization indicated a lack of a chronic effect on the workers (Ermis et al., 2010). In a large study of workers in the pulp and paper industry, exposure to $SO_2$ was associated with increased lung cancer mortality risk compared with unexposed workers; however, the duration of exposure and time since first exposure were not associated with mortality (W. J. Lee et al., 2002). A literature review evaluating evidence of reproductive and developmental effects (Kaufman et al., 2011) found associations with increased incidence of pre-term birth, low birth weight, and other measures of reduced fetal growth when evaluating results from more than 50 studies in humans and 14 in animals. The State of California has listed $SO_2$ among chemicals known to cause reproductive toxicity because of its developmental toxicity (OEHHA, 2011).

Studies of $SO_2$ provided no evidence for identifying specific long-term effects that might be associated with exposure during SHAD testing.

**Trioctyl Phosphate (TOF or TEHP)** [chemical simulant]

TOF is also known as Tris(2-ethylhexyl) phosphate, or TEHP. It is used as a solvent and as a fire retardant or plasticizer for polyvinyl chloride. Exposure to the general population occurs principally via food and drinking water. TOF was used in Project SHAD as a simulant for the chemical warfare nerve agent VX.

Short-term health effects from exposure to TOF appear to be limited. In animals it induces mild temporary irritation of the skin, eye, and respiratory system. A skin test on a small number of human volunteers resulted in redness but no signs of significant skin irritation (WHO, 2000, citing Kimmerle, 1958).

Longer-term studies in animals show a mild chronic inflammation in dogs' lungs after 3 months of regular exposures averaging 85 $mg/m^3$ (WHO, 2000, citing MacFarland and Punte, 1966). This effect was not seen in rhesus monkeys, and no other toxic effect was seen in the testing. Neurotoxicity and cytotoxicity studies have been negative. TEHP did not inhibit cholinesterase. It had a dose-related effect on the trained behavior of dogs but not monkeys (WHO, 2000, citing MacFarland and Punte, 1966). There is no evidence of genotoxicity from tests for sister-chromatid exchanges or chromosomal aberrations, and mutagenicity tests have been negative (CRI, 2004l).

NTP studies carried out in 1984 produced several negative results in tests of carcinogenicity in rats and mice, with the exception of positive findings for liver adenoma and carcinoma in female B6C3F1 mice and phaeochromocytomas in male rats (NTP, 1984). There was a dose-related increase in follicular cell hyperplasia of the thyroid in mice, but no dose-related increase in thyroid tumors (HSDB, 2003b). These findings have not been considered sufficient evidence for concluding that exposure is associated with a significant risk of human carcinogenicity. No studies on potential reproductive effects have been identified.

The search for newer literature on TOF/TEHP identified few studies published since the CRI review (2004l), and the articles that were identified did not provide new information concerning potential long-term health effects from exposure to the compound.

Studies of TEHP provided no evidence for identifying specific long-term health effects that might be associated with exposure during SHAD testing.

**Uranine** [tracer]

Uranine, also known as sodium flourescein, is a dye that is used as a fluorescent tracer in medical and environmental studies. For example, it is regularly used in ophthalmologic procedures to evaluate blood flow. It was used in the SHAD test designated Speckled Start.

The new literature search primarily identified reports related to medical uses of uranine as a tracer or contrast agent. Intravenous administration of uranine is in rare instances associated with anaphylactic shock (e.g., Bearelly et al., 2009) and more commonly with nausea (L. R. Lee et al., 2001). It is also being used in confocal laser endomicroscopy (CLE) of the GI tract. No serious adverse effects were observed in a multicenter study of CLE that included 2,252 patients (Wallace et al., 2010). Localized dermal application of uranine does not appear to be associated with health effects (O'Goshi and Serup, 2006). Only one study (in rats) was identified that was relevant to exposure through inhalation (Sakagami et al., 2003), which is the most likely manner in which the SHAD veterans who participated in the Speckled Start test may have been exposed. In rats that received nose-only inhalation exposures to uranine, absorption occurred in the nasal passages, the lungs, and the GI tract. Of the total absorption, 63.3 percent occurred in the GI tract, 24.2 percent in the nasal passages, and 12.5 percent in the lungs (Sakagami et al., 2003). Another study evaluated oral administration of sodium fluorescein for use in staining part of the eye (the clear vitreous) prior to vitrectomy. No short-term effects were found (Yao et al., 2007).

Studies of uranine provided no evidence for identifying specific long-term health effects that might be associated with exposure during SHAD testing.

**VX** [active chemical nerve agent]

VX is a chemical warfare agent that is an oily viscous liquid. It is an organophosphate compound[4] with a chemical formula of $C_{11}H_{26}NO_2PS$. It exists in several isomers, with CAS registry numbers of 50782-69-9, 51848-47-6, 53800-40-1, and 70938-84-0. Two tests involving releases of VX were reported as part of Project SHAD, one of which involved release over an unmanned barge.

VX is a very potent inhibitor of AChEs, resulting in stimulation of nicotinic, muscarinic, and central nervous system receptors as a result of the buildup of acetylcholine in the synapses of central and peripheral nerves. Acute effects from overstimulation of nicotinic receptors include fatigue, muscle twitching, cramps, and muscle paralysis, including muscles of the respiratory system. Muscarinic effects include miosis, headaches, blurred vision, rhinorrhea, bradycardia, anorexia, nausea, vomiting, diarrhea, sweating, and lacrimation. Acute central nervous system effects are cyanosis, hypotension, generalized weakness, convulsions, loss of consciousness, coma, and death.

The symptoms, severity, and course of toxicity from VX exposure vary by dose and exposure route. When sublethal doses are applied to the skin, hours may elapse before the onset of symptoms. The response to dermal exposure to a small drop of VX may start with localized sweating and muscle twitching, followed by nausea, vomiting, diarrhea, and generalized weakness, typically lasting for several hours. When higher doses of VX are applied to the skin, no symptoms may appear for up to 30 minutes, followed by rapid loss of consciousness, difficulty breathing, convulsions, secretions from nose and mouth, muscle twitching, paralysis,

---

[4] See footnote 3 regarding information related to organophosphate pesticides.

and death. Via dermal exposure, VX is considered at least 100 times more toxic than sarin (CRI, 2004m).

Effects from inhalation of VX typically occur within minutes. Symptoms resulting from exposure to low to moderate concentrations include miosis, rhinorrhea, and airway constriction. Relatively short-lived neuropsychiatric effects, such as loss of memory and depression, are also seen following inhalation of VX. In the absence of medical treatment, larger doses result in loss of consciousness, seizures, cessation of cardiac and respiratory activity, and death. Via inhalation, VX is considered twice as lethal as sarin (CRI, 2004m).

Little is known about the long-term toxicity of VX and other nerve agents. Textbooks indicate that effects dissipate within months after exposure, and "VX exposure has not been shown to have delayed or persistent psychological effects or result in any long-term EEG changes" (CRI, 2004m, p. 4). A telephone survey of volunteers who had participated in military testing of chemical agents found greater sleep disturbances reported by those who had been exposed to nerve agents, and fewer attention problems (Page, 2003). Unlike many other organophosphates, VX has not been shown to induce a syndrome called organophosphorus-induced delayed neuropathy (OPIDN). It has also tested negative in assays for mutagenicity and teratogenicity. It is not considered to be a carcinogen (CRI, 2004m).

The literature search update identified many studies related to VX published since the review carried out for the first SHAD study (CRI, 2004). Most of these newer reports focused on refining understanding of animal models and methods for conducting animal tests (e.g., Aurbeck et al., 2006; Nambiar et al., 2006; Rocksen et al., 2008; Wetherell et al., 2008). Some reports were based on testing done in cell culture systems (e.g., Tenn et al., 2012; Thiermann et al., 2010). Among the reports relevant to potentially lasting effects from sub-lethal exposures to VX was evidence from a study in which rats received months of exposure to low doses of VX through osmotic pumps. Changes in the Open Field test[5] and expression of a certain membrane protein in hippocampal neurons that were evident immediately following termination of exposure had returned to normal after one month (Bloch-Shilderman et al., 2008). Another evaluation of behavioral and biochemical effects in rats of sub-lethal inhalation exposure to VX found only minor performance effects despite substantial biochemical effects (Genovese et al., 2007). A similar experiment with African green monkeys also found that at doses producing substantial inhibition of AChE but no clinical signs, behavioral performance up to 12 weeks after exposure was unaffected (Genovese et al., 2011). In guinea pigs exposed by inhalation to sub-lethal concentrations of VX, changes in respiratory dynamics returned to normal levels by one month following termination of exposure (Rezk et al., 2007).

Studies of VX provided no evidence for identifying specific long-term health effects that might be associated with exposure during SHAD testing.

### Zinc Cadmium Sulfide (ZnCdS) [tracer]

ZnCdS is a compound formed by sintering (combining with heat) zinc sulfide (ZnS) and cadmium sulfide (CdS). It is stable and brightly fluorescent, and it is used in pigments and as a visualization agent. It was used as a tracer for chemical and biological warfare agents in Project SHAD testing.

---

[5] The Open Field Test is an experiment used as a measure of a rodent's movement and willingness to explore, sometimes considered a measure of anxiety (Prut and Belzung, 2003).

ZnCdS was also used as a simulant for biological warfare agents in releases over cities in the United States and the United Kingdom in the 1950s and 1960s. Public concern regarding possible health effects from this testing led to an evaluation by a committee of the National Research Council (NRC, 1997). Although limited information was available on the potential toxicity of ZnCdS, the available data suggested minimal toxicity because the substance is insoluble and unlikely to become bioavailable.

However, the NRC committee carried out a risk assessment using the "worst case" assumption that the ZnCdS broke down into its original components of ZnS and CdS. Under that scenario, CdS is the component of concern because cadmium compounds have been shown to be carcinogenic in humans, with clearest evidence for lung cancer and suggestive evidence for prostate cancer (IARC, 2011). Long-term exposure to cadmium is also harmful to kidney tubules and results in kidney dysfunction. The NRC (1997) risk assessment found that the amount of cadmium to which people might have been exposed in the releases over urban areas was too low to pose a significant health risk. An independent expert assessment carried out on behalf of the United Kingdom came to similar conclusions, noting that "the maximum possible inhaled dose as a result of the Ministry of Defense trials was small relative to background concentrations of inhaled cadmium" (Academy of Medical Sciences, 1999; Elliot et al., 2002, p. 16).

In response to an NRC recommendation for additional research, the Army conducted a study to determine the bioavailability and pulmonary toxicity of ZnCdS in animals (Bergmann et al., 2000). The study found that ZnCdS instilled intratracheally into male Fischer rats at levels 500 to 30,000 times the doses estimated to have been received by residents in the test cities produced insterstitial inflammation and accumulation of foreign material in the lungs and mediastinal lymph nodes. Accumulations of zinc and cadmium in the lungs successively declined at 7 days and 14 weeks after dosing, with indications that the ZnCdS was being cleared from the lungs, mostly within 24 hours of dosing, and was not breaking into elemental components. Small amounts of zinc and cadmium were found in the kidney.

Only one publication that examined potential long-term health effects from ZnCdS exposure was identified as having appeared since the CRI (2004n) review. As one of two case studies used to demonstrate a tool for spatial epidemiological analysis integrating health and environmental data, researchers analyzed the geographic variation in risk of esophageal cancer in relation to ZnCdS exposure in Norwich, United Kingdom (Beale et al., 2010). The standardized risks of esophageal cancer in the county in question were lower than those of England and Wales as a whole, and geographic patterns of rates differed in males and females, suggesting no common geographically determined exposure was likely.

Based on the evidence available regarding potential long-term health effects associated with exposure to ZnCdS, the committee tested the hypotheses that participation in SHAD tests that used this compound may be associated with increased risk for the following conditions:

- Lung cancer
- Kidney disease

## REFERENCES

Academy of Medical Sciences. 1999. *Zinc cadmium sulphide dispersion trials.* London, UK: The Academy of Medical Sciences.

Alshukairi, A. N., M. G. Morshed, and N. E. Reiner. 2006. Q fever presenting as recurrent, culture-negative endocarditis with aortic prosthetic valve failure: A case report and review of the literature. *The Canadian Journal of Infectious Diseases & Medical Microbiology* 17(6):341-344.

Andersson, E., A. Knutsson, S. Hagberg, T. Nilsson, B. Karlsson, L. Alfredsson, and K. Toren. 2006. Incidence of asthma among workers exposed to sulphur dioxide and other irritant gases. *European Respiratory Journal* 27(4):720-725.

Angelakis, E., and D. Raoult. 2010. Q fever. *Veterinary Microbiology* 140(3-4):297-309.

ATSDR (Agency for Toxic Substances and Disease Registry). 2008. *Toxicological profile for phenol.* Atlanta, GA: Agency for Toxic Substances and Disease Registry, Public Health Service, U.S. Department of Health and Human Services.

ATSDR. 2011. *Calcium hypochlorite/sodium hypochlorite.* http://www.atsdr.cdc.gov/substances/toxsubstance.asp?toxid=192 (accessed December 7, 2015).

Aurbek, N., H. Thiermann, L. Szinicz, P. Eyer, and F. Worek. 2006. Analysis of inhibition, reactivation and aging kinetics of highly toxic organophosphorus compounds with human and pig acetylcholinesterase. *Toxicology* 224(1-2):91-99.

Bacci, S., S. Villumsen, P. Valentiner-Branth, B. Smith, K. A. Krogfelt, and K. Molbak. 2012. Epidemiology and clinical features of human infection with *Coxiella burnetii* in Denmark during 2006-07. *Zoonoses and Public Health* 59(1):61-68.

Bachmeyer, C., M. Sanguina, Y. Turc, G. Reynaert, and L. Blum. 2004. Necrotizing fasciitis due to *Serratia marcescens. Clinical and Experimental Dermatology* 29(6):673-674.

Baggish, A. L., and H. Nadiminti. 2007. Intracranial abscess from embolic *Serratia marcescens* endocarditis. *Lancet Infectious Diseases* 7(9):630.

Beale, L., S. Hodgson, J. J. Abellan, S. Lefevre, and L. Jarup. 2010. Evaluation of spatial relationships between health and the environment: The rapid inquiry facility. *Environmental Health Perspectives* 118(9):1306-1312.

Bearelly, S., S. Rao, and S. Fekrat. 2009. Anaphylaxis following intravenous fluorescein angiography in a vitreoretinal clinic: Report of 4 cases. *Canadian Journal of Ophthalmology* 44(4):444-445.

Berger, J., M. Diab-Elschahawi, A. Blacky, E. Pernicka, V. Spertini, O. Assadian, W. Koller, and K. J. Aichberger. 2010. A matched prospective cohort study on *Staphylococcus aureus* and *Escherichia coli* bloodstream infections: Extended perspectives beyond resistance. *American Journal of Infection Control* 38(10):839-845.

Bergmann, J. D., L. W. Metker, W. C. McCain, P. A. Beall, M. W. Michie, and R. B. Lee. 2000. Intratracheal instillation of zinc-cadmium sulfide (ZnCdS) in Fischer 344 rats. *Inhalation Toxicology* 12(4):331-346.

Bloch-Shilderman, E., I. Rabinovitz, I. Egoz, L. Raveh, N. Allon, E. Grauer, E. Gilat, and B. A. Weissman. 2008. Subchronic exposure to low-doses of the nerve agent VX: Physiological, behavioral, histopathological and neurochemical studies. *Toxicology and Applied Pharmacology* 231(1):17-23.

Bruce, W., M. E. Meek, and R. Newhook. 2001. Phenol: Hazard characterization and exposure-response analysis. *Journal of Environmental Science and Health, Part C: Environmental Carcinogenesis and Ecotoxicology Reviews* 19(1):305-324.

CCRIS (Chemical Carcinogenesis Research Information System). 2010. *Methyl acetoacetate.* http://toxnet.nlm.nih.gov/newtoxnet/ccris.htm (accessed December 7, 2015).

CDC (Centers for Disease Control and Prevention). 2011. *Q fever.* http://www.cdc.gov/qfever (accessed December 7, 2015).

CDC. 2012. *Statistics and epidemiology: Annual cases of Q fever in the United States.* http://www.cdc.gov/qfever/stats/index.html (accessed December 7, 2015).

CIDRAP (Center for Infectious Disease Research and Policy). 2010. *Tularemia.* http://www.cidrap.umn.edu/cidrap/content/bt/tularemia/biofacts/tularemiafactsheet.html#_Overview_1+CIDRAP (accessed December 7, 2015).

Clark Burton, N., A. Adhikari, S. A. Grinshpun, R. Hornung, and T. Reponen. 2005. The effect of filter material on bioaerosol collection of *Bacillus subtilis* spores used as a *Bacillus anthracis* simulant. *Journal of Environmental Monitoring* 7(5):475-480.

CRI (Center for Research Information). 2004a. *Health effects of Project SHAD biological agent: Bacillus globigii.* Silver Spring, MD: Center for Research Information, Inc.

CRI. 2004b. *Health effects of Project SHAD biological agent: Coxiella burnetii.* Silver Spring, MD: Center for Research Information, Inc.

CRI. 2004c. *Health effects of Project SHAD biological agent: Pasteurella [Francisella] tularensis.* Silver Spring, MD: Center for Research Information, Inc.

CRI. 2004d. *Health effects of Project SHAD biological agent: Serratia marcescens.* Silver Spring, MD: Center for Research Information, Inc.

CRI. 2004e. *Health effects of Project SHAD biological agent: Staphylococal enterotoxin type B.* Silver Spring, MD: Center for Research Information, Inc.

CRI. 2004f. *Health effects of Project SHAD chemical agent: Betapropiolactone.* Silver Spring, MD: Center for Research Information, Inc.

CRI. 2004g. *Health effects of Project SHAD chemical agent: Calcofluor.* Silver Spring, MD: Center for Research Information, Inc.

CRI. 2004h. *Health effects of Project SHAD chemical agent: Diethylphthalate.* Silver Spring, MD: Center for Research Information, Inc.

CRI. 2004i. *Health effects of Project SHAD chemical agent: Methyl acetoacetate.* Silver Spring, MD: Center for Research Information, Inc.

CRI. 2004j. *Health effects of Project SHAD chemical agent: Sarin nerve agent.* Silver Spring, MD: Center for Research Information, Inc.

CRI. 2004k. *Health effects of Project SHAD chemical agent: Sulfur dioxide.* Silver Spring, MD: Center for Research Information, Inc.

CRI. 2004l. *Health effects of Project SHAD chemical agent: Trioctyl phosphate.* Silver Spring, MD: Center for Research Information, Inc.

CRI. 2004m. *Health effects of Project SHAD chemical agent: VX nerve agent.* Silver Spring, MD: Center for Research Information, Inc.

CRI. 2004n. *Health effects of Project SHAD chemical agent: Zinc cadmium sulfide.* Silver Spring, MD: Center for Research Information, Inc.

Cullu, E., I. Ozkan, N. Culhaci, and B. Alparslan. 2005. A comparison of the effect of doxorubicin and phenol on the skeletal muscle. May doxorubicin be a new alternative treatment agent for spasticity? *Journal of Pediatric Orthopaedics, Part B* 14(2):134-138.

Dennis, D. T., T. V. Inglesby, D. A. Henderson, J. G. Bartlett, M. S. Ascher, E. Eitzen, A. D. Fine, A. M. Friedlander, J. Hauer, M. Layton, S. R. Lillibridge, J. E. McDade, M. T. Osterholm, T. O'Toole, G. Parker, T. M. Perl, P. K. Russell, and K. Tonat. 2001. Tularemia as a biological weapon–Medical and public health management. *Journal of the American Medical Association* 285(21):2763-2773.

DoD (Department of Defense). 2002. *Fact sheet: DTC test 68-50.* http://www.health.mil/Reference-Center/Fact-Sheets/2002/05/23/DTC-Test-6850 (accessed December 7, 2015).

Dokic, M., M. Milanovic, V. Begovic, A. Ristic-Andelkov, and B. Tomanovic. 2004. Infective endocarditis of a rare etiology (*Serratia marcescens*). [Croatian]. Vojnosanitetski Pregled. *Military-Medical and Pharmaceutical Review* 61(6):689-694.

DTC (Deseret Test Center). 1968. *DTC test 66-13 (Half Note).* Fort Douglas, UT: Deseret Test Center.

Duncan, E. J. S., B. Kournikakis, J. Ho, and I. Hill. 2009. Pulmonary deposition of aerosolized *Bacillus atrophaeus* in a Swine model due to exposure from a simulated anthrax letter incident. *Inhalation Toxicology* 21(2):141-152.

Elliott, P. J., C. J. C. Phillips, B. Clayton, and P. J. Lachmann. 2002. The risk to the United Kingdom population of zinc cadmium sulfide dispersion by the Ministry of Defence during the "cold war." *Occupational and Environmental Medicine* 59(1):13-17.

Ermis, H., M. Gokirmak, Z. Yildirim, S. Yologlu, and H. Ankarali. 2010. Exposure to SO2 does not have a chronic effect on pulmonary functions of apricot workers. *Inhalation Toxicology* 22(3):219-223.

EurActiv. 2004. *EU ministers agree to ban chemicals in toys.* http://www.euractiv.com/health/eu-ministers-agree-ban-chemicals-news-212475 (accessed December 7, 2015).

Fraser, J. D. 2011. Clarifying the mechanism of superantigen toxicity. *PLoS Biology* 9(9):e1001145. doi:10.1371/journal.pbio.1001145.

Friedman, N. D., N. B. Peterson, W. T. Sumner, and B. D. Alexander. 2003. Spontaneous dermal abscesses and ulcers as a result of *Serratia marcescens. Journal of the American Academy of Dermatology* 49(2 Suppl Case Reports):S193-S194.

Friend, J. C., D. M. Hilligoss, M. Marquesen, J. Ulrick, T. Estwick, M. L. Turner, E. W. Cowen, V. Anderson, S. M. Holland, and H. L. Malech. 2009. Skin ulcers and disseminated abscesses are characteristic of *Serratia marcescens* infection in older patients with chronic granulomatous disease. *Journal of Allergy and Clinical Immunology* 124(1):164-166.

Geier, D. A., S. K. Jordan, and M. R. Geier. 2010. The relative toxicity of compounds used as preservatives in vaccines and biologics. *Medical Science Monitor* 16(5):SR21-SR27.

Genovese, R. F., B. J. Benton, E. H. Lee, S. J. Shippee, and E. M. Jakubowski. 2007. Behavioral and biochemical evaluation of sub-lethal inhalation exposure to VX in rats. *Toxicology* 232(1-2):109-118.

Genovese, R. F., B. J. Benton, J. L. Oubre, C. E. Byers, E. M. Jakubowski, R. J. Mioduszewski, T. J. Settle, and T. J. Steinbach. 2011. Determination of threshold adverse effect doses of percutaneous VX exposure in African green monkeys. *Toxicology* 279(1-3):65-72.

Goktepe, S., M. Kilic, S. Gunduz, R. Alaca, and T. A. Kalyon. 2002. The effect of botulinum toxin and phenol injections on lower extremity spasticity in spinal cord injury. *Journal of Rheumatology and Medical Rehabilitation* 13(2):113-117.

Gray, L. E., Jr., J. Ostby, J. Furr, M. Price, D. N. Veeramachaneni, and L. Parks. 2000. Perinatal exposure to the phthalates DEHP, BBP, and DINP, but not DEP, DMP, or DOTP, alters sexual differentiation of the male rat. *Toxicological Sciences* 58(2):350-365.

Hartzell, J. D., R. N. Wood-Morris, L. J. Martinez, and R. F. Trottta. 2008. Q fever: Epidemiology, diagnosis, and treatment. *Mayo Clinic Proceedings* 83(5):574-579.

Healy, B., H. van Woerden, D. Raoult, S. Graves, J. Pitman, G. Lloyd, N. Brown, and M. Llewelyn. 2011. Chronic Q fever: Different serological results in three countries—Results of a follow-up study 6 years after a point source outbreak. *Clinical Infectious Diseases* 52(8):1013-1019.

Henderson, R. F., E. B. Barr, W. B. Blackwell, C. R. Clark, C. A. Conn, R. Kalra, T. H. March, M. L. Sopori, Y. Tesfaigzi, M. G. Menache, and D. C. Mash. 2002. Response of rats to low levels of sarin. *Toxicology and Applied Pharmacology* 184(2):67-76.

HSDB (Hazardous Substances Data Bank). 2003a. *Phenol.* http://toxnet.nlm.nih.gov/cgi-bin/sis/search2/f?./temp/~sB4HnY:1 (accessed December 7, 2015).

HSDB. 2003b. *Trioctyl phosphate.* http://toxnet.nlm.nih.gov/cgi-bin/sis/search2/f?./temp/~3CRU19:1 (accessed December 7, 2015).

HSDB. 2005. *Methyl acetoacetate.* http://toxnet.nlm.nih.gov/cgi-bin/sis/search2/f?./temp/~atmJKb:1 (accessed December 7, 2015).

Huang, C. R., C. H. Lu, C. C. Chien, and W. N. Chang. 2001. Protean infectious types and frequent association with neurosurgical procedures in adult *Serratia marcescens* CNS infections: Report of two cases and review of the literature. *Clinical Neurology and Neurosurgery* 103(3):171-174.

Hume, E. B. H., and M. D. P. Willcox. 2004. Emergence of *Serratia marcescens* as an ocular surface pathogen. *Archivos de la Sociedad Espanola de Oftalmologia* 79(10):475-477.

IARC (International Agency for Research on Cancer). 1992. *Occupational exposures to mists and vapours from strong inorganic acids; and other industrial chemicals.* IARC Monographs Vol. 54. Lyon, France: World Health Organization. Pp. 131-188.

IARC. 1997. *Chlorinated drinking-water; chlorination by-products; some other halogenated compounds; cobalt and cobalt compounds.* IARC Monographs Vol. 52. Lyon, France: World Health Organization. Pp. 7-10.

IARC. 1999a. *Re-evaluation of some organic chemicals, hydrazine and hydrogen peroxide: β-propiolactone.* IARC Monographs Vol. 71. Lyon, France: World Health Organization. Pp. 1103-1119.

IARC. 1999b. *Re-evaluation of some organic chemicals, hydrazine and hydrogen peroxide: Phenol.* IARC Monographs Vol. 71. Lyon, France: World Health Organization. Pp. 749-768.

IARC. 2011. *Cadmium and cadmium compounds.* IARC Monographs Vol. 100C. Lyon, France: World Health Organization. Pp. 121-145.

Iglesias, M. E. L., J. V. De Cabo, J. T. Traspaderne, J. A. Franco, M. B. Alonso, and R. B. De Bengoa Vallejo. 2008. Safety of phenol vapor inhalation during performance of chemical matrixectomy to treat ingrown toenails. *Dermatologic Surgery* 34(11):1515-1519.

IOM (Institute of Medicine). 2000. *Gulf war and health, volume one: Depleted uranium, sarin, pyridostigmine bromide, and vaccines.* Washington, DC: National Academy Press.

IOM. 2003. *Gulf war and health, volume two: Insecticides and solvents.* Washington, DC: The National Academies Press.

IOM. 2004. *Gulf war and health: Updated literature review of sarin.* Washington, DC: The National Academies Press.

IOM. 2007a. *Gulf War and health, volume five: Infectious diseases.* Washington, DC: The National Academies Press.

IOM. 2007b. *Long-term health effects of participation in Project SHAD (Shipboard Hazard and Defense).* Washington, DC: The National Academies Press.

Jarrett, L., P. Nandi, and A. J. Thompson. 2002. Managing severe lower limb spasticity in multiple sclerosis: Does intrathecal phenol have a role? *Journal of Neurology, Neurosurgery and Psychiatry* 73(6):705-709.

Kaminaka, C., Y. Yamamoto, N. Yonei, and F. Furukawa. 2009a. Phenol application to angiosarcomas: Implications and histologic studies. *International Journal of Dermatology* 48(5):470-475.

Kaminaka, C., Y. Yamamoto, N. Yonei, A. Kishioka, T. Kondo, and F. Furukawa. 2009b. Phenol peels as a novel therapeutic approach for actinic keratosis and bowen disease: Prospective pilot trial with assessment of clinical, histologic, and immunohistochemical correlations. *Journal of the American Academy of Dermatology* 60(4):615-625.

Kampschreur, L. M., S. Dekker, J. Hagenaars, P. J. Lestrade, N. H. M. Renders, M. G. L. de Jager-Leclercq, M. H. A. Hermans, C. A. R. Groot, R. H. H. Groenwold, A. I. M. Hoepelman, P. C. Wever, and J. J. Oosterheert. 2012. Identification of risk factors for chronic Q fever, the Netherlands. *Emerging Infectious Diseases* 18(4):563-570.

Kaufman, F. L., A. N. Kim, M. A. Campbell, K. L. Wu, and J. M. Donald. 2011. *Sulfur dioxide-evidence of reproductive and developmental toxicity.* Birth Defects Research Part A—Clinical and Molecular Teratology Conference: 51st Annual Meeting of the Teratology Society—24th International Conference of the Organization of Teratology Information Specialists, OTIS and the 35th Annual Meeting of the Neurobehavioral Teratology Society, NBTS Coronado, CA. Conference Publication: (var. pagings) 91(5):378.

Kawada, T., M. Katsumata, H. Suzuki, Q. Li, H. Inagaki, A. Nakadai, T. Shimizu, K. Hirata, and Y. Hirata. 2005. Insomnia as a sequela of sarin toxicity several years after exposure in Tokyo subway trains. *Perceptual and Motor Skills* 100(3 Pt 2):1121-1126.

Kelly, A. R., F. W. Hartman, and C. E. Rupe. 1957. The toxicology of beta-propiolactone. In *Hepatitis Frontiers*, edited by F. W. Hartman, G. A. LoGrippo, J. G. Mateer, and J. Barron. Boston, MA: Little, Brown and Company. Pp. 387-406.

Kimber, I., and R. J. Dearman. 2010. An assessment of the ability of phthalates to influence immune and allergic responses. *Toxicology* 271 (3):73-82.

Kimmerle, G. 1958. *[Softener tri-2-ethylhexylphosphate (TOF).]* Unpublished report No. 1764 (in German). Leverkusen, Germany: Bayer AG, Laboratory of Toxicology and Pathology.

Kolaski, K., S. J. Ajizian, L. Passmore, N. Pasutharnchat, L. A. Koman, and B. P. Smith. 2008. Safety profile of multilevel chemical denervation procedures using phenol or botulinum toxin or both in a pediatric population. *American Journal of Physical Medicine and Rehabilitation* 87(7):556-566.

Kwack, S. J., K. B. Kim, H. S. Kim, and B. M. Lee. 2009. Comparative toxicological evaluation of phthalate diesters and metabolites in Sprague-Dawley male rats for risk assessment. *Journal of Toxicology and Environmental Health Part A: Current Issues* 72(21-22):1446-1454.

Langrock, M. L., H. J. Linde, M. Landthaler, and S. Karrer. 2008. Leg ulcers and abscesses caused by *Serratia marcescens*. *European Journal of Dermatology* 18(6):705-707.

Lee, J. H., Y. T. Lin, Y. H. Yang, L. C. Wang, and B. L. Chiang. 2005. Increased levels of serum-specific immunoglobulin e to staphylococcal enterotoxin A and B in patients with allergic rhinitis and bronchial asthma. *International Archives of Allergy and Immunology* 138(4):305-311.

Lee, L. R., D. P. Hainsworth, C. W. Hamm, and R. W. Madsen. 2001. Temperature effect on nausea during fluorescein angiography. *Ophthalmology* 108(7):1193-1195.

Lee, W. J., K. Teschke, T. Kauppinen, A. Andersen, P. Jappinen, I. Szadkowska-Stanczyk, N. Pearce, B. Persson, A. Bergeret, L. A. Facchini, R. Kishi, D. Kielkowski, B. A. Rix, P. Henneberger, J. Sunyer, D. Colin, M. Kogevinas, and P. Boffetta. 2002. Mortality from lung cancer in workers exposed to sulfur dioxide in the pulp and paper industry. *Environmental Health Perspectives* 110(10):991-995.

Li, R., and Z. Meng. 2007. Effects of $SO_2$ derivatives on expressions of MUC5AC and IL-13 in human bronchial epithelial cells. *Archives of Toxicology* 81(12):867-874.

Li, R., Z. Meng, and J. Xie. 2007a. Effects of sulfur dioxide derivatives on four asthma-related gene expressions in human bronchial epithelial cells. *Toxicology Letters* 175(1-3):71-81.

Li, R., Z. Meng, and J. Xie. 2007b. Effects of sulfur dioxide on the expressions of MUC5AC and ICAM-1 in airway of asthmatic rats. *Regulatory Toxicology and Pharmacology* 48(3):284-291.

Li, R., Z. Meng, and J. Xie. 2008. Effects of sulfur dioxide on the expressions of EGF, EGFR, and COX-2 in airway of asthmatic rats. *Archives of Environmental Contamination and Toxicology* 54(4):748-757.

Liangpunsakul, S., and K. Pursell. 2001. Community-acquired necrotizing fasciitis caused by *Serratia marcescens*: Case report and review. *European Journal of Clinical Microbiology and Infectious Diseases* 20(7):509-510.

Liu, T., B. Q. Wang, and P. C. Yang. 2006a. A possible link between sinusitis and lower airway hypersensitivity: The role of staphylococcal enterotoxin B. *Clinical and Molecular Allergy* 4:7.

Liu, T., B.-Q. Wang, P.-Y. Zheng, S.-H. He, and P.-C. Yang. 2006b. Rhinosinusitis derived staphylococcal enterotoxin B plays a possible role in pathogenesis of food allergy. *BMC Gastroenterology* 6:24.

LoGrippo, G. A. 1964. A ten year clinical study of plasma treated with betaprone and combined bataprone plus ultraviolet irradiation. *Pacific Medicine and Surgery* 72:298-302.

MacFarland, H. N., and C. L. Punte, Jr. 1966. Toxicological studies on tri-(2-ethylhexyl)-phosphate. *Archives of Environmental Health* 13(1):13-20.

Mah-Sadorra, J. H., D. M. Najjar, C. J. Rapuano, P. R. Laibson, and E. J. Cohen. 2005. *Serratia* corneal ulcers: A retrospective clinical study. *Cornea* 24(7):793-800.

Mahajan, R., A. Blair, C. F. Lynch, P. Schroeder, J. A. Hoppin, D. P. Sandler, and M. C. Alavanja. 2006. Fonofos exposure and cancer incidence in the Agricultural Health Study. *Environmental Health Perspectives* 114(2):1838-1842.

Mahlen, S. D. 2011. *Serratia* infections: From military experiments to current practice. *Clinical Microbiology Reviews* 24(4):755-791.

Meng, Z., and B. Zhang. 2002. Induction effects of sulfur dioxide inhalation on chromosomal aberrations in mouse bone marrow cells. *Mutagenesis* 17(3):215-217.

Meng, Z., G. Qin, B. Zhang, H. Geng, Q. Bai, W. Bai, and C. Liu. 2003. Oxidative damage of sulfur dioxide inhalation on lungs and hearts of mice. *Environmental Research* 93(3):285-292.

Meng, Z., G. Qin, B. Zhang, and J. Bai. 2004. DNA damaging effects of sulfur dioxide derivatives in cells from various organs of mice. *Mutagenesis* 19(6):465-468.

Meng, Z., G. Qin, and B. Zhang. 2005. DNA damage in mice treated with sulfur dioxide by inhalation. *Environmental and Molecular Mutagenesis* 46(3):150-155.

Mills, P. K., and R. Yang. 2003. Prostate cancer risk in California farm workers. *Journal of Occupational and Environmental Medicine* 45(3):249-258.

Miyaki, K., Y. Nishiwaki, K. Maekawa, Y. Ogawa, N. Asukai, K. Yoshimura, N. Etoh, Y. Matsumoto, Y. Kikuchi, N. Kumagai, and K. Omae. 2005. Effects of sarin on the nervous system of subway workers seven years after the Tokyo subway sarin attack. *Journal of Occupational Health* 47(4):299-304.

Munro, N. B., K. R. Ambrose, and A. P. Watson. 1994. Toxicity of the organophosphate chemical warfare agents GA, GB, and VX: Implications for public protection. *Environmental Health Perspectives* 102:18-38.

Nambiar, M. P., B. S. Wright, P. E. Rezk, K. B. Smith, R. K. Gordon, T. S. Moran, S. M. Richards, and A. M. Sciuto. 2006. Development of a microinstillation model of inhalation exposure to assess lung injury following exposure to toxic chemicals and nerve agents in guinea pigs. *Toxicology Mechanisms and Methods* 16(6):295-306.

NIOSH (National Institute for Occupational Safety and Health). 2011. *NIOSH skin notation (SK) profiles: Phenol.* Publication No. 2011-136. Atlanta, GA: National Institute for Occupational Safety and Health, Centers for Disease Control and Prevention, U.S. Department of Health and Human Services.

NRC (National Research Council). 1997. *Toxicologic assessment of the Army's zinc cadmium sulfide dispersion tests.* Washington, DC: National Academy Press.

NTP (National Toxicology Program). 1984. *NTP toxicology and carcinogenesis studies of tris(2-ethylhexyl)phosphate (CAS No. 78-42-2) in F344/N rats and B6C3F1 mice (gavage studies).* National Toxicology Program Technical Report Series 274. Triangle Park, NC: U.S. Department of Health and Human Services, Public Health Service, National Toxicology Program.

NTP. 2011. *Report on carcinogens, Twelfth ed.* Research Triangle Park, NC: U.S. Department of Health and Human Services, Public Health Service, National Toxicology Program. Pp. 366-367.

OEHHA (California Office of Environmental Health Hazard Assessment). 2011. *Sulfur dioxide listed to cause reproductive toxicity.* http://oehha.ca.gov/prop65/prop65_list/072911list2.html (accessed December 7, 2015).

O'Goshi, K., and J. Serup. 2006. Safety of sodium fluorescein for in vivo study of skin. *Skin Research and Technology* 12(3):155-161.

Pereira, C., K. Mapuskar, and C. V. Rao. 2006. Chronic toxicity of diethyl phthalate in male Wistar rats—A dose-response study. *Regulatory Toxicology and Pharmacology* 45(2):169-177.

Pereira, C., K. Mapuskar, and C. V. Rao. 2007. Chronic toxicity of diethyl phthalate—A three generation lactational and gestational exposure study on male Wistar rats. *Environmental Toxicology and Pharmacology* 23(3):319-327.

Pikhart, H., M. Bobak, P. Gorynski, B. Wojtyniak, J. Danova, M. A. Celko, B. Kriz, D. Briggs, and P. Elliott. 2001. Outdoor sulphur dioxide and respiratory symptoms in Czech and Polish school children: A small-area study (SAVIAH). Small-area variation in air pollution and health. *International Archives of Occupational and Environmental Health* 74(8):574-578.

Pinder, C., B. Bhakta, and K. Kodavali. 2008. Intrathecal phenol: An old treatment revisited. *Disability and Rehabilitation* 30(5):381-386.

Probst, A., R. Facius, R. Wirth, and C. Moissl-Eichinger. 2010. Validation of a nylon-flocked-swab protocol for efficient recovery of bacterial spores from smooth and rough surfaces. *Applied and Environmental Microbiology* 76(15):5148-5158.

Prut, L., and C. Belzung. 2003. The open field as a paradigm to measure the effects of drugs on anxiety-like behaviors: A review. *European Journal of Pharmacology* 463(1-3):3-33.

Rajagopalan, G., M. M. Sen, M. Singh, N. S. Murali, K. A. Nath, K. Iijima, H. Kita, A. A. Leontovich, U. Gopinathan, R. Patel, and C. S. David. 2006a. Intranasal exposure to staphylococcal enterotoxin B elicits an acute systemic inflammatory response. *Shock* 25(6):647-656.

Rajagopalan, G., M. K. Smart, R. Patel, and C. S. David. 2006b. Acute systemic immune activation following conjunctival exposure to staphylococcal enterotoxin B. *Infection and Immunity* 74(10):6016-6019.

Raoult, D. , H. Tissot-Dupont, C. Foucault, J. Gouvernet, P. E. Fournier, E. Bernit, A. Stein, M. Nesri, J. R. Harle, and P. J. Weiller. 2000. Q fever 1985-1998: Clinical and epidemiologic features of 1,383 infections. *Medicine* 79(2):109-123.

Raoult, D., T. Marrie, and J. Mege. 2005. Natural history and pathophysiology of Q fever. *The Lancet Infectious Diseases* 5(4):219-226.

Rezk, P. E., J. R. Graham, T. S. Moran, R. K. Gordon, A. M. Sciuto, B. P. Doctor, and M. P. Nambiar. 2007. Acute toxic effects of nerve agent VX on respiratory dynamics and functions following microinsillation inhalation exposure in guinea pigs. *Inhalation Toxicology* 19(3):291-302.

Rocksen, D., D. Elfsmark, V. Heldestad, K. Wallgren, G. Cassel, and A. Goransson Nyberg. 2008. An animal model to study health effects during continuous low-dose exposure to the nerve agent VX. *Toxicology* 250(1):32-38.

Rusnak, J. M., M. Kortepeter, R. Ulrich, M. Poli, and E. Boudreau. 2004. Laboratory exposures to staphylococcal enterotoxin B. *Emerging Infectious Diseases* 10(9):1544-1549.

Sakagami, M., W. Kinoshita, and Y. Makino. 2003. Fractional contribution of lung, nasal and gastrointestinal absorption to the systemic level following nose-only aerosol exposure in rats: A case study of 3.7-micro m fluorescein aerosols. *Archives of Toxicology* 77(6):321-329.

Sang, N., L. Hou, Y. Yun, and G. Li. 2009. SO(2) inhalation induces protein oxidation, DNA-protein crosslinks and apoptosis in rat hippocampus. *Ecotoxicology and Environmental Safety* 72(3):879-884.

Sang, N., Y. Yun, H. Li, L. Hou, M. Han, and G. Li. 2010. $SO_2$ inhalation contributes to the development and progression of ischemic stroke in the brain. *Toxicological Sciences* 114(2):226-236.

Sang, N., Y. Yun, G. Y. Yao, H. Y. Li, L. Guo, and G. K. Li. 2011. $SO_2$-induced neurotoxicity is mediated by cyclooxygenases-2-derived prostaglandin e-2 and its downstream signaling pathway in rat hippocampal neurons. *Toxicological Sciences* 124(2):400-413.

Sanz-Garcia, M., A. Fernandez-Cruz, M. Rodriguez-Creixems, E. Cercenado, M. Marin, P. Munoz, and E. Bouza. 2009. Recurrent *Escherichia coli* bloodstream infections: Epidemiology and risk factors. *Medicine* 88(2):77-82.

Smith, J. L., and D. Bayles. 2007. Postinfectious irritable bowel syndrome: A long-term consequence of bacterial gastroenteritis. *Journal of Food Protection* 70(7):1762-1769.

Soria, X., I. Bielsa, M. Ribera, M. J. Herrero, H. Domingo, J. M. Carrascosa, and C. Ferrandiz. 2008. Acute dermal abscesses caused by *Serratia marcescens*. *Journal of the American Academy of Dermatology* 58(5):891-893.

Tenn, C. C., M. T. Weiss, C. Beaup, A. Peinnequin, Y. Wang, and F. Dorandeu. 2012. Cyclooxygenase-2 contributes to VX-induced cell death in cultured cortical neurons. *Toxicology Letters* 210(1):71-77.

Thiermann, H., T. Seeger, S. Gonder, N. Herkert, B. Antkowiak, T. Zilker, F. Eyer, and F. Worek. 2010. Assessment of neuromuscular dysfunction during poisoning by organophosphorus compounds. *Chemico-Biological Interactions* 187(1-3):265-269.

Tomi, N. S., B. Kranke, and E. Aberer. 2005. Staphylococcal toxins in patients with psoriasis, atopic dermatitis, and erythroderma, and in healthy control subjects. *Journal of the American Academy of Dermatology* 53(1):67-72.

van der Hoek, W., P. M. Schneeberger, T. Oomen, M. C. Wegdam-Blans, F. Dijkstra, D. W. Notermans, H. A. Bijlmer, K. Groeneveld, C. J. Wijkmans, A. Rietveld, L. M. Kampschreur, and Y. van Duynhoven. 2012. Shifting priorities in the aftermath of a Q fever epidemic in 2007 to 2009 in the Netherlands: From acute to chronic infection. *Eurosurveillance* 17(3):16-20

Wallace, M. B., A. Meining, M. I. Canto, P. Fockens, S. Miehlke, T. Roesch, C. J. Lightdale, H. Pohl, D. Carr-Locke, M. Lohr, E. Coron, B. Filoche, M. Giovannini, J. Moreau, C. Schmidt, and R. Kiesslich. 2010. The safety of intravenous fluorescein for confocal laser endomicroscopy in the gastrointestinal tract. *Alimentary Pharmacology and Therapeutics* 31(5):548-552.

Wen, Y. K. 2012. Necrotizing fasciitis caused by *Serratia marcescens*: A fatal complication of nephrotic syndrome. *Renal Failure* 34(5):649-652.

Wetherell, J. R., S. J. Armstrong, R. W. Read, and G. F. Clough. 2008. VX penetration following percutaneous poisoning: A dermal microdialysis study in the guinea pig. *Toxicology Mechanisms and Methods* 18(4):313-321.

WHO (World Health Organization). 2000. *Environmental health criteria 218: Flame retardants: Tris(2-butoxyethyl)phosphate, tris(2-ethylhexyl)phosphate and tetrakis(hydroxymethyl)phosphonium salts.* Geneva, Switzerland: United Nations Environment Programme, the International Labour Organisation, and the World Health Organization.

WHO. 2003. *Concise international chemical assessment document, 52: Diethyl phthalate.* Geneva, Switzerland: United Nations Environment Programme, the International Labour Organization, and the World Health Organization.

Yamasue, H., O. Abe, K. Kasai, M. Suga, A. Iwanami, H. Yamada, M. Tochigi, T. Ohtani, M. A. Rogers, T. Sasaki, S. Aoki, T. Kato, and N. Kato. 2007. Human brain structural change related to acute single exposure to sarin. *Annals of Neurology* 61(1):37-46.

Yanagisawa, N., H. Morita, and T. Nakajima. 2006. Sarin experiences in Japan: Acute toxicity and long-term effects. *Journal of the Neurological Sciences* 249(1):76-85.

Yao, Y., Z.-J. Wang, S. H. Wei, Y. F. Huang, and M. N. Zhang. 2007. Oral sodium fluorescein to improve visualization of clear vitreous during vitrectomy for proliferative diabetic retinopathy. *Clinical and Experimental Ophthalmology* 35(9):824-827.

Yoshida, R., Y. Takae, Y. Fujio, M. Tanaka, and M. Ohyama. 2009. Cutaneous *Serratia marcescens* infection on the face of a healthy female. *Journal of the European Academy of Dermatology and Venereology* 23(10):1213-1215.

Yoshihiro, Y., Y. Soejima, K. Taniguchi, K. Makino, and S. Naito. 2010. A case of *Serratia* granuloma in the soft tissue around the left kidney: A role of PTHrP in the formation of *Serratia* granuloma. *Journal of Infection and Chemotherapy* 16(2):126-130.

Zhang, J., C. Liang, J. Ma, B. Zhou, and J. Wang. 2006a. Changes in testis protein and metabolic enzyme activities in rats induced by sodium fluoride and sulfur dioxide. *Fluoride* 39(3):179-184.

Zhang, J., C. Liang, J. Ma, B. Zhou, and J. Wang. 2006b. Effects of sodium fluoride and sulfur dioxide on oxidative stress and antioxidant defenses in rat testes. *Fluoride* 39(3):185-190.

Ziemann, C., T. Hansen, G. Pohlmann, D. Farrar, C. Pohlenz-Michel, and I. Mangelsdorf. 2009. *Absence of genotoxicity of sulfur dioxide ($SO_2$) in a bone marrow micronucleus test with NMRI mice, complemented with several hematological endpoints.* Toxicology Letters Conference: 46th Congress of the European Societies of Toxicology, EUROTOX 2009 Dresden Germany. Conference Publication: (var. pagings) 189:S258.

# Appendix D

# Additional Information on Data and Methods Used for Analysis

This appendix supplements Chapters 3, 4, and 5 with additional detail on specific features of the data used in the study and the analyses that were performed. The supplemental discussion of study data focuses on the process used to gather data on cause of death among the members of the study population, particularly those who died before 1979; the choice of health outcomes to be used as endpoints in the analyses; the approach used to represent the likely variation among the veterans of the Shipboard Hazard and Defense (SHAD) tests in exposure to test substances and potential exposure modifiers; and the selection of comparison groups to be used in the analyses of health outcomes in populations of special interest. Additional detail on the study's analyses addresses the selection of analyses to perform; Kaplan-Meier and Cox regression models for survival data, including consideration of competing risks and ship-clustering in analyses of specific causes of death; and correction for multiple comparisons.

## DATA CONSIDERATIONS

### Ascertainment of Cause of Death

*Deaths from 1979 Through 2011*

Information on deaths that have occurred in the United States since January 1979 can be obtained from the National Death Index (NDI). NDI is operated by the National Center for Health Statistics (NCHS, 2015) and is a compilation of information from death certificates issued by states. A service called NDI Plus provides the codes from the *International Classification of Diseases* (ICD) (WHO, 2015) for the underlying cause of death as indicated on the death certificate. The codes are assigned in accordance with the version of the ICD in use at the time the death occurred.

A total of 4,068 men in the study population were identified as having died by December 31, 2011, which was the conclusion of the follow-up period. Of these deaths, 2,357 occurred between January 1, 1979, and December 31, 2004, and were included in the SHAD I study (IOM, 2007). The information on cause of death that was gathered from NDI for the SHAD I study was used again in the SHAD II study.

Of the other deaths in the study population, 1,334 were men identified as having died between January 1, 2005, and December 31, 2011. Information on the cause of death was obtained directly from NDI Plus. Criteria for identifying a match between a record in the SHAD database and a record in the NDI database were agreement on all nine digits of the social security number, first and last name, and date of birth. The cause-of-death information was received in electronic form. No information on cause of death was obtained for 175 of the 3,694 deaths that occurred between 1979 and the end of December 2011.

*Deaths Before 1979*

In the study population 374 deaths are recorded as having occurred before January 1, 1979. Of these, cause of death was identified for 191 and was not for 184. Identifying the causes of these "early" deaths required determining the state in which the person died and submitting a request to the state's vital records office for a copy of the death certificate. However, place of death is not reliably recorded in the study population's records from the Department of Veterans Affairs (VA) and the Department of Defense (DoD). And when a place of death is known, each state has its own procedures and requirements for processing requests for death certificates. For the SHAD I study it did not prove feasible to undertake the collection of death certificates from individual states. As a result, that study included analyses of the timing of deaths but not the causes of pre-1979 deaths.

For the SHAD II study, an effort was made to obtain information on the causes of as many of these early deaths as possible. To identify the states where the deaths had occurred information from deceased veterans' VA and DoD records on residence and claims processing was supplemented with searches of electronic death indexes maintained by some states and other online genealogic resources that provide information about date, location, and in a few cases, cause of death.

Requests for death certificates were submitted to 34 states, the District of Columbia, and the Philippines, resulting in the receipt of 184 death certificates from 28 states. Death certificates were received from the states of Arizona, California, Colorado,[1] Connecticut, Florida,[2] Georgia, Hawaii, Illinois, Indiana, Kentucky, Louisiana, Maryland,[3] Michigan, Minnesota, Mississippi, Missouri,[4] Nebraska, New Jersey, North Carolina, Ohio, Oregon, Pennsylvania, South Carolina, Tennessee,[5] Utah, Virginia, Washington, and Wisconsin. Requests were also submitted to Alabama, Arizona, the District of Columbia, Massachusetts, Nevada, the Philippines, and Rhode Island; but the requested death certificates were not located. The procedures to obtain access to

---

[1] These data were supplied by the Health Statistics Section of the Colorado Department of Public Health and Environment, which specifically disclaims responsibility for any analyses, interpretations, or conclusions it has not provided.

[2] The Florida Department of Health is acknowledged for their contribution of data. Conclusions are those of the authors and do not necessarily reflect the opinion of the Florida Department of Health.

[3] Certain data were provided by the Vital Statistics administration, Maryland Department of Health and Mental Hygiene, Baltimore, Maryland. The Department of Health and Mental Hygiene disclaims responsibility for any analyses, interpretations, or conclusions.

[4] Some of the data used in this report was acquired from the Missouri Department of Health and Senior Services (DHSS). The contents of this document, including data analysis, interpretation, or conclusions are solely the responsibility of the authors and do not represent the official views of DHSS.

[5] Vital records data were provided by the Tennessee Department of Health, Division of Policy, Planning, and Assessment, Office of Health Statistics.

death records were not successfully completed for deaths thought to have occurred in Iowa, New York, Oklahoma, and Texas. Death certificates were not sought from the states of Alaska, Delaware, Idaho, Kansas, Maine, Montana, New Hampshire, North Dakota, South Dakota, Vermont, West Virginia, or Wyoming because there were no indications that early deaths in the SHAD study population had occurred there.

Upon receipt of a death certificate from a state, the dates of death and birth were compared with the information in the study's database to confirm that match was correct. For confirmed matches, a study case number was assigned to the death certificate. Identifying information was redacted, and the redacted document was sent to a nosologist who coded the underlying cause of death according to the ninth and tenth revisions of the ICD. The nosologist had no knowledge of whether the decedent was a SHAD test participant or a member of the comparison group.

Other online sources produced information on the causes of an additional 14 early deaths. These sources included the Combat Area Casualties Current File, which provided information for 13 of these deaths. The Combat Area Casualties Current File hold final records of service members who died in Southeast Asia or are listed as missing in action from 1956 through 1998 (National Archives, 2015). The records were updated as of December 1998. A search of the U.S. Find A Grave Index (Tipton, 2015) produced information on the cause for the other death in this group. Information on the causes of these 14 deaths was sent to the nosologist for ICD coding.

## Choice of Study Endpoints

Because a large number of health outcomes (e.g., deaths from various causes, inpatient or outpatient care for various illnesses) could be investigated for possible association with SHAD exposure, the committee used two approaches to guide its work. One approach was hypothesis-driven and the other was considered exploratory.

### *Hypothesis-Driven Selection of Health Outcomes*

As described in the main body of the report and in Appendix C, the committee undertook a review of recent literature to identify adverse health outcomes that might be associated with exposure to substances used in the SHAD tests. This review resulted in the identification of six substances for which the published literature suggested a basis for proposing hypotheses that exposure could be associated with increased risk of certain adverse health outcomes (see Table D-1).

### *Health Outcomes for Exploratory Analysis*

In addition to examining the health outcomes suggested by the literature review, the committee sought to examine the data for signals of any other effects that might not have been anticipated based on individual exposures, but could have resulted from the particular combinations or circumstances of the testing. For this, the committee chose to examine mortality and morbidity in broad ICD-9 (and ICD-10 for mortality) categories. In addition, the committee included a category of neurocognitive disease (ICD-9: 290-319, 320-327; ICD-10: F00-99, G00-09) because memory and attention scores from the health questionnaire used in the SHAD I study had indicated greater problems among participants than controls (IOM, 2007, p. 56).

**TABLE D-1** Hypotheses to Be Tested Concerning Certain Substances Used in SHAD Testing and Adverse Health Outcomes

| Substance | Use in SHAD Test | Health Outcome Hypothesized |
| --- | --- | --- |
| *Coxiella burnetii* | Biological agent | Chronic hepatitis<br>Endocarditis<br>Fatigue syndrome<br>Osteomyelitis<br>Vascular infection |
| *Escherichia coli* | Biological simulant | Irritable bowel syndrome |
| Staphylococcal enterotoxin type B[a] | Biological agent | Asthma<br>Graves' disease<br>Multiple sclerosis<br>Rheumatoid arthritis (broad or narrow definition) |
| Sarin | Chemical agent | Neurological effects (central nervous system)<br>Neurological effects (peripheral nervous system)<br>Neurological effects (hearing loss)<br>Psychological symptoms |
| Betapropiolactone | Decontaminant | Cancer (any type) |
| Zinc cadmium sulfide | Tracer | Chronic kidney disease (broad or narrow definition)<br>Lung cancer |

[a] Because the individuals who served on the vessels involved in testing staphylococcal enterotoxin type B were not identified, the committee could not test the hypotheses generated for this agent.

## REPRESENTATION OF POTENTIAL EXPOSURE LEVELS

As described in Chapter 3, the committee considered exposure in terms of the substances used in SHAD tests and number of times each SHAD participant had the potential to be exposed to a substance. The number of trials for which an individual was present during each test and the total number of potential exposure opportunities for a given test substance over all tests were used as indicators of exposure. The distribution of exposure opportunities was plotted for each individual test substance and for exposures to any biological agent, any chemical agent (except trioctyl phosphate), and any decontaminant.

The plots informed decisions as to whether and how to group the participants into distinct exposure subgroups to facilitate group comparisons and analysis of potential exposure dose-response relationships. This subgrouping was done only when the number of men in the exposure group was large enough to ensure that each subgroup was greater than 100 in size. In environmental epidemiology and research in health-related fields, grouping subjects according to levels of exposure or other risk factors is common. The principle is that subgrouping would reach a balance between maximal similarity among individuals within a subgroup and maximal distinction across subgroups with respect to important characteristics and implied health risk (O'Brien, 2004). In the absence of knowledge of associated health risk, subgrouping is done with respect to one or more selected characteristics of the participants. The distribution of SHAD exposures was not continuous, often had multiple clusters (modes) because the participants assigned to the same ship were more likely to have similar numbers of exposures (see Figure D-1), or skewed with a small number of individuals having a larger number of exposures (see Figure D-2). These features rendered the conventional subgrouping schemes such as tertiles, quartiles, or equal length less useful because they could more likely fail to differentiate between subgroups or fail to homogenize within a subgroup.

For exposure to betapropriolactone, the quantile approach would lead to three groups: 1-2 exposures, 3-8 exposures, and 9 exposures. In this case, the second group is dominated by 8 exposures (101/123), hardly different from the third subgroup. These observations invited different approaches to subgrouping.

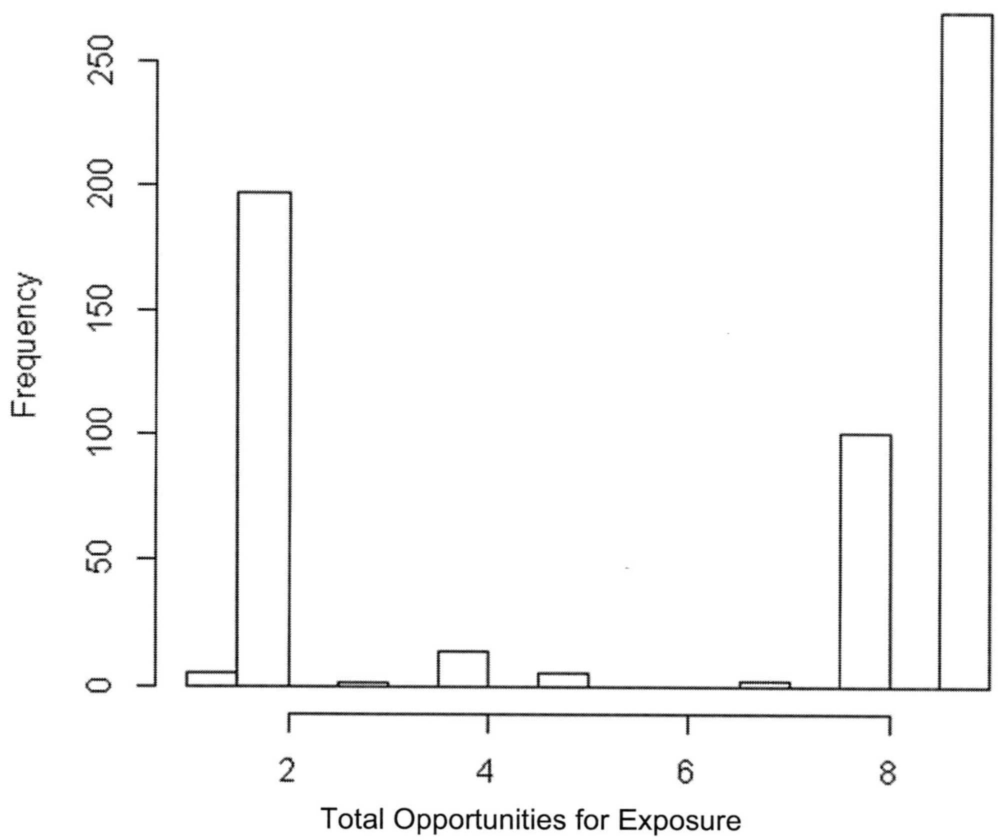


**FIGURE D-1** Frequency distribution of SHAD veterans' total number of opportunities for exposure to betapropiolactone (BPL). With this distribution, two groups are formed: lower (1-5 exposure opportunities n = 222) and higher (6-9 exposure opportunities, n = 373). The boundary is half the distance between the two modes (2 exposures and 9 exposures). Exposure opportunities are releases of the test substances on or over the ship or unit.

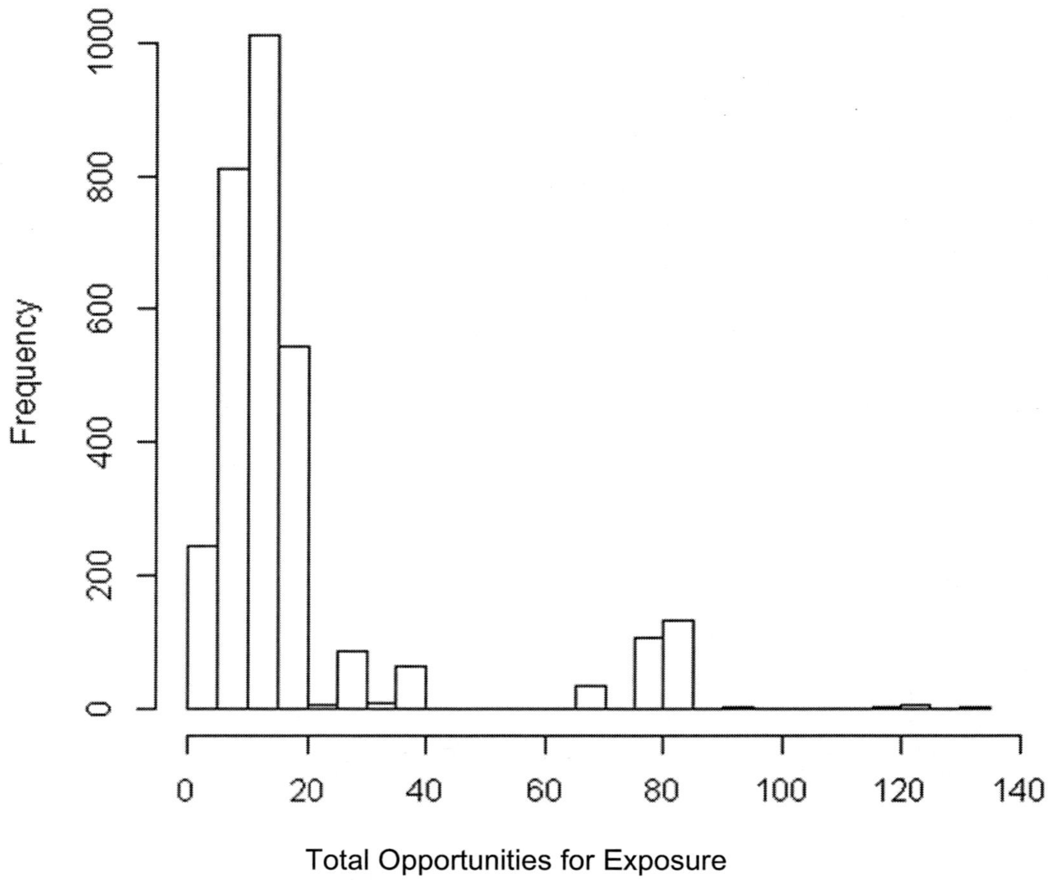


**FIGURE D-2** Frequency distribution of SHAD veterans' total number of opportunities for exposure to any of the chemical substances used in SHAD tests, except trioctyl phosphate (TOF). The skewness is greater than three, so the quartile approach was used. The participants were broken into four equal groups. The first three groups were combined to make up the lower group (1-20 exposure opportunities, n = 1,812), and the upper quartile made up the higher group (≥21 exposure opportunities, n = 724). Exposure opportunities are releases of the test substances on or over the ship or unit.

Thus, the modes (clusters) and percentiles of the number of exposure opportunities were determined using the routine "density" in R (version 3.0.3) for kernel estimation. The modes and percentiles together define exposure groups as described below in detail. Use of the algorithm resulted in two to three subgroups depending on the shape of the distribution and the number of participants involved in that exposure condition. The algorithm is as follows:

1. If the total number of participants was less than 400, do not subdivide. (These were mostly cases where the number of exposure opportunities was clustered around one mode [ship]).
2. If the total number of participants was more than 400, determine modes of the distribution (using kernel estimation with a bandwidth of 1/10 or 1/20 of the range of potential exposures [Sheather and Jones, 1991]).
   2a. If there are multiple modes,
      a. Determine the midpoints between the neighboring modes and use these middle values as grouping cutoff points.
      b. If any subgroup has fewer than 100 members, combine it with its nearest neighbor of smaller group size.
   2b. If there is only one mode, 2 groups will be formed as follows:
      a. If skewness is less than 3 in absolute value, the tertiles approach was used with the first 2/3 of the values forming one group and the remaining 1/3 the other group.
      b. If skewness is greater than 3, the quartile approach was used with the first 3/4 of the participants used in forming the first group and the last 1/4 the second group.

Ships were the experimental units in the SHAD tests, and individuals were exposed in clusters by ships. Such a clustering structure should ideally be retained in forming the exposure subgroups.

Thus for betapropiolactone, two modes were identified as shown in Figure D-1. For individuals with exposures to any of the chemical substances, there was only one mode (see Figure D-2) and the approach described in 2b.b. above was used to identify two groupings.

## GROUPS OF SPECIAL INTEREST

### USS *George Eastman*, USS *Granville S. Hall*, and the Light Tugs

Most of the participants in SHAD testing were involved in only one test, and most tests made use of a simulant in place of an active biological or chemical agent. However, both the USS *George Eastman* and the light tugs were involved not only in tests that used simulants, but also in tests that used active chemical or biological agents. For various tests of both types, the USS *Granville S. Hall* served as a laboratory ship that was to be kept clear of the dispersal of the test agents. However, its laboratory staff handled and analyzed samples collected by others during and after the tests. To allow for the special features of their SHAD experiences, the committee examined the health outcomes for the crew of the USS *George Eastman* and the light tug boats and other Project SHAD technical staff (PSTS), including the laboratory staff on the USS *Granville S. Hall*, separately from other SHAD participants in some analyses.

For the seven tests the USS *George Eastman* participated in over 1963-1966, two different ships served as comparisons. The USS *Interceptor* was the comparison ship for the tests Eager Belle I, Eager Belle II, Errand Boy, Flower Drum I, and Magic Sword, and the USS *Oxford* for tests Fearless Johnny and Half Note.

Identification of an appropriate comparison group was more difficult for the PSTS who served aboard the five light tugs and as laboratory and meteorological staff aboard the USS

*Granville S. Hall*. As noted in Chapter 2, the tugs had been Army tugs that were modified to include a laboratory "doghouse" and to be resistant to air leaks to the interior (Testimony to IOM Committee on Shipboard Hazard and Defense, February 2012). The tug crews and PSTS were specially assigned to the tugs or to the USS *Granville S. Hall*, and were required to hold Secret or Top Secret security clearance. Moreover, the men who served as PSTS have been explicitly identified for only one test, Shady Grove, except for a handful who stepped forward and were confirmed by DoD to have served on the tugs.

Given these challenges, two approaches were used to designate a comparison group for the tug crews and other PSTS. One comparison group (internal control) was the crew on the USS *Granville S. Hall* who were not part of the PSTS. These crew members were present on the USS *Granville S. Hall*, but they were not allowed to cross a clear boundary into the sample handling/laboratory area. The alternative comparison group (external control) was the crew on the ship named as the comparison ship for the USS *Granville S. Hall* for a given test (Shady Grove).

## DATA ANALYSIS

### Analyses for Mortality

Kaplan-Meier survival curves were used for a first, "crude," comparison of the number and timing of deaths in the participant and comparison groups. Changes in mortality over time in the two groups may not be at a constant rate. The Kaplan-Meier comparison takes these and other data features into consideration and is capable of detecting a persistent difference in mortality over time. It is not, however, adjusted for group difference due to age and other important risk factors. For example, all other risk factors being equal, a population that is older will experience earlier mortality than a younger population, which is reflected in a more rapidly descending line representing the proportion of the older group still alive at a given time point.

Cox proportional hazard regression analysis was also used. It takes the Kaplan-Meier comparison a step further to incorporate individuals' exposure and other risk factors such as age into consideration. It can also take into consideration data clustering at the ship level. Use of the proportional hazards model assumes proportionality in the associated hazard functions (force of mortality). Proportionality was confirmed graphically by plotting the logarithm of cumulative hazard based on Kaplan-Meier estimates versus the logarithm of time. Cox proportional hazard regression was used to assess all-cause mortality and cause-specific mortality for the overall study population and for the exposure groups examined.

The model was fitted in two ways. For the unadjusted model, mortality was the outcome and only participant or comparison status was used as the explanatory variable. For the adjusted models, participant and comparison status or in some instances the number of exposure opportunities was the main exposure variable; age and rank (enlisted versus officer) were also included as explanatory variables. Service branch (Navy versus Marines and other) was included as an explanatory variable for analyses of the overall study population and the analysis of TOF exposure, which included a larger proportion of Marine participants. Because of the large amount of missing data on the race of the SHAD participants and comparison population and the lack of a feasible way to impute the missing data, the committee decided not to include race in the analysis. The committee did not observe differential exposure by race and had no reason to anticipate a differential effect of exposure based on race. In many cases, the analysis was stratified by officer and enlisted status in order to see if officers and enlisted personnel had a different mortality experience. When the exposed and comparison groups included personnel from multiple ships,[6] data clustering at the ship level was considered, which described both a possible data correlation among individuals on the same ship as well as potential differences between the ships. In all analyses, a variable designating the ship to which a person was assigned during the test was used in the model as a random effect to quantify ship-clustering. In some instances the estimation process failed to converge with an estimate of the variance for the random effects.

For cause-specific mortality, competing risk was incorporated in the Cox regression model. Death due to the specified cause was considered as the main outcome, and death due to other causes was considered in the model as the outcome of a competing risk.

The committee carried out exploratory analyses involving multiple exposure groups among the SHAD participants that were created using the data grouping described in the previous section. The committee used Cox regression models to explore potential dose-response relationships between exposure level and mortality in conjunction with other factors such as age and enlisted status. SAS (version 9.4) was used for most data analysis, including survival analyses of mortality data. The SAS procedures used were PHREG for Cox regression, NPAR1WAY for Wilcoxon comparisons, LIFETEST for Kaplan-Meier, and FREQUENCY for the Fisher's exact test. For group comparison of rates or proportions, R software was used (as indicated in tables presenting results of analyses) for the Fisher's exact test (using the routine fisher.test) or logistic regressions (using the routine glm), As noted above, kernel density estimation was done in R with the routine density.

## Analyses for Morbidity

The analysis of morbidity compared the SHAD participants and the comparison population on the basis of hospital days (as a measure of general significant morbidity) and of incidence of a diagnosis of a specific disease or disease group. Logistic regression with over-dispersion was used to compare levels of enrollment in Medicare (see Table 5-1), or use of Veterans Health Administration (VHA) medical services (see Table 5-2). The overall enrollment (Medicare) or use (VHA) numbers were compared with the Fisher's exact test. The Fisher's exact test was also used to compare percentages of SHAD participants and members of the comparison groups with a diagnosis code of interest in Tables 5-4, 5-5, 5-6, 5-7, and 5-9. Median hospital days per person-years in Medicare among those with hospitalization claims through Medicare (see Tables 5-3 and 5-8) were compared using a Wilcoxon rank sum test.

Circumstances did not permit the committee to take advantage of the more quantitative metrics of individual level of exposure and available factors to adjust for the heterogeneity in risk among the study participants.

## Additional Statistical Considerations

Testing a large number of exposure-outcome associations increases the chance of reporting spurious associations. In the case of testing a single association at a 0.05 type I error

---

[6] The term "ship" should be understood to mean the military unit to which a person was assigned at the time of a given SHAD test. For the majority of the study population, the unit was a ship, but some men were assigned to aviation or infantry units.

level, approximately 5 percent of observed, significant associations would be the result of chance alone when there is no such association. When there are m distinct associations to be tested independently, each at a 5 percent error level, the family-wise error rate (FWER) of reporting at least one false association when there is none increases to $1-(1-0.05)^m \approx m*0.05-m*(m-1)/2*0.05^2+\ldots$. To control FWER at 5 percent, for example, the Bonferroni correction essentially divides m into the 5 percent nominal level to form an adjusted nominal level of significance, and a test whose p-value is less than the adjusted significance level would be declared to be significant. The Holm's correction divides the sequence of m, m–1, …, into the 5 percent nominal level to form adjusted nominal levels of significance for the tests ascending from the smallest to largest p-value; tests with a p-value less than their respective adjusted significance level are significant.

Because the multiple tests in the analysis of SHAD data, in particular those involving the same exposure and comparison groups, are less likely to be independent and because the adjustment to control FWER could compromise the ability to report a true significant test, the committee adopted the false discovery rate (FDR) correction. The FDR considers the percentage of false significant tests among all significant tests. The Benjamini and Hochberg (1995) adjustment multiplies the overall FDR rate level (e.g., 5 percent) by j/m as the nominal significance level for the test with the jth smallest p-value; a test with a p-value less than its corresponding nominal level is significant. The committee chose to use this FDR adjustment when any test reached an unadjusted nominal level of 5 percent.

The committee applied the Benjamini and Hochberg adjustment to the FDR in two instances in the analyses described in this report. In the analyses reported in Table 4-13, the results showed a statistically significant increase in the hazard ratio for heart disease mortality for the crew of the USS *George Eastman.* The p-values were 0.017 and 0.022, respectively, for models of pooled SHAD participants and of enlisted personnel only. The committee considered FDR adjustment of a multiplicity of three tests associated with cancer, heart diseases, and respiratory diseases in the case of enlisted and officers combined and the case of enlisted only. To retain an overall 0.05 FDR, the nominal level of significance is 0.05*1/3 = 0.0167. Because the observed p-values were greater than 0.0167, they did not reach the significance level. Note that the FDR adjustment for the case with the smallest p-value is the same as the Bonferroni adjustment. Further, the multiplicity of tests would be six if the tests of officers and enlisted together are combined with the enlisted only tests in one set, nine if those with the tugs and Project SHAD technical staff group were included, and would be 41 if the tests with other exposure groups were included, making the observed difference of the USS *George Eastman* crew much less significant.

A second circumstance in which the committee applied the Benjamini and Hochberg adjustment to the FDR to account for the multiple tests carried out was with the results of the analyses presented in Table 5-7. If one considers 10 tests to have been carried out for Table 5-7, then to retain an overall 0.05 FDR, the nominal levels of significance are 0.05*1/10 = 0.005, 0.05*2/10, 0.05*3/10, 0.05*4/10, and 0.05*5/10 for the five tests with p-values less than 0.05 in ascending order. Only the four tests with the smallest p-values reached their respective adjusted nominal level.

The committee did not pursue the few results in which members of the SHAD test participant groups had statistically significantly lower hazard or median hospital days per person-year of Medicare enrollment than members of the comparison groups. The statistical significance was the result of the implicit two-sided alternatives involved in these tests. Under a one-sided alternative of worse outcomes for the SHAD participants, which is the a priori hypothesis of this investigation, these tests would not yield a significant p-value.

The committee considered statistical power in planning the analysis. Based on the data reported in SHAD I (IOM, 2007), statistical power assessment was conducted under various scenarios of the size of the differences, data variation, and error rate to be controlled. In general, a group size of 400 is required to retain a power greater than 65 percent. Given that none of the results of mortality analysis reached a statistical significance level after adjusting for multiple comparisons, the committee determined a post-hoc assessment of power for individual cases to be unnecessary.

The committee was also guided by the requirements of the Centers for Medicare & Medicaid Services (CMS) that prevent reporting of small cell sizes to prevent the identification of any individual. In keeping with the CMS requirements and to take similar precautions with other health outcome data, the committee did not report cell sizes ≤10. In addition, the committee reported only confidence intervals, not point estimates, when there was the potential to back-calculate the number of cases in a small cell. NR, for "not reported," was used in a cell when the results of a calculation were suppressed for this reason.

## Additional Analytical Challenges for Mortality and Morbidity

The committee took a precautionary approach to the overall analysis. Specifically, the use of alternative and supplementary methods aimed to ensure the internal validity as well as the robustness of each analysis.

The committee discussed possible data analytic approaches, such as propensity score matching, to control for confounding effects—differences among the comparison and exposure groups could have affected both the health outcomes and the SHAD exposure. Neither data from the SHAD I report nor data from the SHAD II analysis revealed significant differences between the exposed and comparison groups with respect to demographics and risk factors such as Vietnam experience or life style factors. Further, with the exception of specially outfitted ships such as the USS *George Eastman*, the USS *Granville S. Hall*, the tugs, and the USS *Herbert J. Thomas*, no evidence suggested that the ships participating in the SHAD testing were chosen for reasons that could disqualify other ships that were chosen for the comparison group. The strategy was to investigate bias issues on a case-to-case basis when such a need arose for a specific endpoint.

Investigation of special groups of participants (e.g., those on the tugs, the USS *Granville S. Hall*, and the USS *George Eastman*) remained difficult primarily because the number of people was small. The committee took two alternative and supplementary approaches. One was to compare a special group with its own control despite its small group size. A planned second approach was to include them or exclude them as a form of sensitivity analysis of the specific health endpoint for all participants with the exposure to the same substances.

## Accounting for Location Aboard Ship

An analysis in which differences in exposure are represented by presence during a trial involves the underlying assumption that everyone serving on a test ship was equally at risk for exposure to a test substance. However, it is possible that the potential for exposure was different in different parts of a ship. There are no records of where particular personnel were located during the tests, but the committee envisioned as part of its analysis consideration of the possible impact of a sailor's "job" on his location on or movement about the ship during a test. This aspect of the analysis was not carried out but the nature of this contemplated component of analysis is described here.

The quarterly ship rosters that were used to ascertain who was serving on the ship at the time of the SHAD test (BuPers Report 1080-14) provided information on the pay grade and occupational qualifications (ratings) of the enlisted Navy personnel and the duties to which they were assigned (a "distribution" rating) on that vessel. The committee, with advice from a consultant,[7] assigned crew members to one of three categories or "bins": (1) likely movement around the ship (greater chance of exposure), (2) probable/possible movement, and (3) unlikely movement (less chance of exposure). Special consideration was also given to personnel who were likely to have been assigned to the engine room or the boiler room of a ship. In these areas ventilation requirements may have allowed for an exposure to test agents that did not occur elsewhere on a ship. The committee's designations were made on the basis of typical duties of a person with that rating (Department of the Navy, 2015). The committee knew, however, that during SHAD tests and trials, personnel may have been assigned to locations or duties that were different from their usual assignments.

In addition, the Marines in Test 69-10, who were sprayed with the simulant TOF during a beach landing, were considered to have a potential for exposure equivalent to that of personnel most likely to move about a ship. For officers and personnel in other service branches, the committee judged that rank alone did not provide information about a plausible location or movement during the tests and envisioned using analytic methods to assess the impact of various presumptions about their potential for exposure to test substances.

## Quantitative Exposure Metrics

Quantitative exposure metrics were planned and explored in this study to capture varying degrees of exposure among the SHAD participants to provide an additional dimension for exploring whether an underlying exposure-response relationship exists. The metrics comprise three factors: the types of test agents used in the SHAD tests, the number of trials a person participated in and the number of exposure opportunities he had, and his assigned position (or bin) on the ship. The number of exposure opportunities and bin both provided a more quantitative representation of a person's potential exposure. A categorical score such as 1, 2, and 3 for different bins would give the possibility of ordinal implication. For each test substance or class of substances, the committee considered the number of exposure opportunities and the bin as two separate metrics that would be included in the model both individually and simultaneously, with or without interaction between them. This approach would have allowed investigation of the impact of a metric individually, without or without adjustment to the other, or of a possible synergistic effect of both. Alternatively, if the bins were to demonstrate unequivocal ordinal trend in their impact, they could be used as a "weight" to be combined with the number of exposure opportunities (trials) to form a composite exposure metric. The metrics for individual test substances could also be utilized simultaneously in a model to capture the potential of synergistic effect of a person's cumulative exposure to multiple substances. This could be done in a couple of different ways. One is to include the metrics for the individual

[7] The consultant for this task served in the U.S. Navy for 25 years, retiring in 1981 as a Commander. He served on destroyer escorts, destroyers, and guided missile destroyers in capacities of first lieutenant, weapons officer, operations officer, and executive officer.

substances simultaneously in the model. Another is to sum up relevant individual metrics to form a composite metric especially for similar substances, and include this composite metric in the analysis. The quantitative exposure metrics were planned for use in analyses of both mortality and morbidity. However, because of study circumstances, the use of quantitative exposure metrics described in this section, including the analysis of the possible impact of location on the ship, was not carried out.

## REFERENCES

Benjamini, Y., and Y. Hochberg. 1995. Controlling the false discovery rate: A practical and powerful approach to multiple testing. *Journal of the Royal Statistical Society: Series B* 57(1):289-300.

CDC (Centers for Disease Control and Prevention). 2013. *Classification of diseases, functioning, and disability*. http://www.cdc.gov/nchs/icd.htm (accessed October 13, 2015).

Department of the Navy. 2015. *Manual of Navy enlisted manpower and personnel classifications and occupational standards.* Vol. I, Navy enlisted classifications (NECs). NAVPERS 18068F. Washington, DC. http://www.public.navy.mil/bupers-npc/reference/nec/NECOSVol1/Documents/NAVPERS_18068_FINAL_JUL15.pdf (accessed October 6, 2015).

IOM (Institute of Medicine). 2007. *Long-term health effects of participation in Project SHAD (Shipboard Hazard and Defense).* Washington, DC: The National Academies Press.

National Archives. 2015. *Records of U.S. military casualties, missing in action, and prisoners of war from the era of the Vietnam War.* http://www.archives.gov/research/military/vietnam-war/electronic-records.html (accessed January 31, 2015).

NCHS (National Center for Health Statistics). 2015. *National Death Index.* http://www.cdc.gov/nchs/ndi.htm (accessed October 13, 2015).

O'Brien, S. M. 2004. Cutpoint selection for categorizing a continuous predictor. *Biometrics* 60: 504-509.

Sheather, S. J., and M. C. Jones. 1991. A reliable data-based bandwidth selection method for kernel density estimation. *Journal of the Royal Statistical Society: Series B* 53:683-690.

Tipton, J. 2015. Find a grave. http://www.findagrave.com/cgi-bin/fg.cgi?page=listFaqs#10 (accessed March 24, 2015).

WHO (World Health Organization). 2015. *International Classification of Diseases (ICD).* http://www.who.int/classifications/icd/en (accessed August 4, 2015).

# Appendix E

## Units Participating in Project SHAD Tests and Units Selected as Unexposed Comparisons

**TABLE E-1** Military Units That Participated in Project SHAD Tests and Units Selected as Unexposed Comparisons, by Test

| Participant Unit (hull number) | Unit Type | Operating Area | Comparison Unit (hull number) | Unit Type | Operating Area |
|---|---|---|---|---|---|
| *Autumn Gold (Test 63-2)* | | | | | |
| USS *Granville S. Hall* (YAG-40) | Auxiliary ship | Pearl Harbor | USS *Interceptor* (AGR-8) | Radar picket ship | Canada, California, Portland |
| USS *Navarro* (APA-215) | Attack transport | Pearl Harbor | USS *Talladega* (APA-208) | Attack transport | Long Beach |
| USS *Tioga County* (LST-1158) | Tank landing ship | Pearl Harbor | USS *Vernon County* (LST-1161) | Tank landing ship | Japan, Philippines |
| USS *Carpenter* (DD-825) | Destroyer | Pearl Harbor | USS *John R. Craig* (DD-885) | Destroyer | San Diego |
| USS *Hoel* (DDG-13) | Guided missile destroyer | Pearl Harbor | USS *Towers* (DDG-9) | Guided missile destroyer | San Diego |
| Marine Air Group 13, VMA 214 | Attack squadron | — | Marine Air Group 14, VMA 332 | Attack squadron | — |
| *Big Tom (Test 65-6)* | | | | | |
| USS *Granville S. Hall* (YAG-40) | Auxiliary ship | Pearl Harbor | USS *Oxford* (AGTR-1) | Auxiliary ship | Philippines |
| USS *Carbonero* (SS-337) | Submarine | Hawaii | USS *Raton* (SS-270) | Submarine | San Clemente, San Diego |
| *Copper Head (Test 65-1)* | | | | | |
| USS *Power* (DD-839) | Destroyer | — | USS *Gyatt* (DD-712) | Destroyer | Virginia |
| *DTC Test 69-10* | | | | | |
| USS *Fort Snelling* (LSD-30) | Dock landing ship | — | USS *Spiegel Grove* (LSD-32) | Dock landing ship | Virginia, North Carolina, Puerto Rico |
| Landing Force Carib 1-69/BLT, 1st Battalion, 8th Marines, 2nd Marine Division | Infantry | — | 1st Battalion, 6th Marines, 2nd Marine Division | Infantry | — |
| VMA 324, MAG-32 | Attack squadron | — | VMA 324, MAG-32 | Attack squadron | — |
| *DTC Test 69-31* | | | | | |
| USS *Herbert J. Thomas* | Destroyer | Pearl Harbor | USS *Agerholm* | Destroyer | San Diego |

| Participant Unit (hull number) | Unit Type | Operating Area | Comparison Unit (hull number) | Unit Type | Operating Area |
|---|---|---|---|---|---|
| (DD-833) | | | (DD-826) | | |
| *DTC Test 69-32* | | | | | |
| USS *Granville S. Hall* (YAG-40) | Auxiliary ship | Pearl Harbor | USS *Jamestown* (AGTR-3) | Auxiliary ship | Philippines, South China Sea, Thailand, Vietnam, Special Operations |
| Five light tugs (hull numbers not specified) | — | — | None selected | — | — |
| *Eager Belle I (Test 63-1)* | | | | | |
| USS *George Eastman* (YAG-39) | Auxiliary ship | Pearl Harbor and maneuvers | USS *Interceptor* (AGR-8) | Radar picket ship | San Francisco Picket Stations 1 and 9 |
| *Eager Belle II (Test 63-1)* | | | | | |
| USS *George Eastman* (YAG-39) | Auxiliary ship | Pearl Harbor | USS *Interceptor* (AGR-8) | Radar picket ship | San Francisco Picket Stations 1, 3, 9 |
| USS *Tioga County* (LST-1185) | Tank landing ship | Pearl Harbor | USS *Vernon County* (LST-1161) | Tank landing ship | Hong Kong, Japan, Okinawa, Taiwan |
| USS *Carpenter* (DD-825) | Destroyer | Pearl Harbor | USS *Agerholm* (DD-826) | Destroyer | Hong Kong, Japan, Okinawa, Philippines |
| USS *Granville S. Hall* (YAG-40) | Auxiliary ship | — | USS *Interdictor* (AGR-13) | Radar picket ship | — |
| USS *Navarro* (APA-215) | Attack transport | — | USS *Noble* (APA-218) | Attack transport | — |
| Marine Medium Helicopter Squadron 161 | — | — | Marine Medium Helicopter Squadron 161 | — | — |
| *Errand Boy (Test 64-1)* | | | | | |
| USS *George Eastman* (YAG-39) | Auxiliary ship | Pearl Harbor | USS *Interceptor* (AGR-8) | Radar picket ship | San Francisco, Picket Station 7 |
| *Fearless Johnny (Test 65-17)* | | | | | |
| USS *George Eastman* (YAG-39) | Auxiliary ship | — | USS *Oxford* (AGTR-1) | Auxiliary ship | Hong Kong, Philippines |
| USS *Granville S. Hall* (YAG-40) | Auxiliary ship | Pearl Harbor | USS *Georgetown* (AGTR-2) | Auxiliary ship | Hong Kong, Philippines |

| Participant Unit (hull number) | Unit Type | Operating Area | Comparison Unit (hull number) | Unit Type | Operating Area |
|---|---|---|---|---|---|
| *Flower Drum I (Test 64-2)* | | | | | |
| USS *George Eastman* (YAG-39) | Auxiliary ship | Pearl Harbor | USS *Interceptor* (AGR-8) | Radar picket ship | San Francisco, San Diego, Radar Picket Stations 1, 5, 7 |
| USS *Granville S. Hall* (YAG-40) | Auxiliary ship | — | USS *Interdictor* (AGR-13) | Radar picket ship | — |
| *Folded Arrow (Test 68-71)* | | | | | |
| USS *Granville S. Hall* (YAG-40) | Auxiliary ship | Pearl Harbor | USS *Oxford* (AGTR-1) | Auxiliary ship | Philippines, South China Sea |
| USS *Carbonero* (SS-337) | Submarine | Pearl Harbor | USS *Tunny* (SS-282) | Submarine | Philippines, Special Operations |
| Five light tugs (hull numbers not specified) | — | — | None selected | — | — |
| *Half Note (Test 66-13)* | | | | | |
| USS *George Eastman* (YAG-39) | Auxiliary ship | — | USS *Oxford* (AGTR-1) | Auxiliary ship | Hong Kong, Taiwan, Special Operations |
| USS *Granville S. Hall* (YAG-40) | Auxiliary ship | Pearl Harbor | USS *Jamestown* (AGTR-3) | Auxiliary ship | Malaysia, Taiwan, Special Operations |
| USS *Carbonero* (SS-337) | Submarine | — | USS *Tunny* (SS-282) | Submarine | Pearl Harbor, Philippines |
| Light tugs 2080, 2081, 2085, 2086, 2087 | — | — | None selected | — | — |
| *High Low (Test 65-13)* | | | | | |
| USS *Berkeley* (DDG-15) | Destroyer | — | USS *Lynde McCormick* (DDG-8) | Destroyer | Hong Kong, Japan, San Diego |
| USS *Fechteler* (DD-870/DDR-870) | Destroyer | — | USS *John R. Craig* (DD-885) | Destroyer | San Diego |
| USS *Okanogan* (APA-220) | Attack transport | — | USS *Montrose* (APA-212) | Attack transport | San Diego, Pearl Harbor, San Clemente |
| USS *Wexford County* (LST-1168) | Tank landing ship | — | USS *Washoe County* (LST-1165) | Tank landing ship | Japan, Okinawa |

| Participant Unit (hull number) | Unit Type | Operating Area | Comparison Unit (hull number) | Unit Type | Operating Area |
|---|---|---|---|---|---|
| *Magic Sword (Test 65-4)* | | | | | |
| USS *George Eastman* (YAG-39) | Auxiliary Ship | Pearl Harbor | USS *Interceptor* (AGR-8) | Auxiliary ship | Durban, Philippines |
| *Purple Sage (Test 66-5_* | | | | | |
| USS *Herbert J. Thomas* (DD-833) | Destroyer | — | USS *Agerholm* (DD-826) | Destroyer | San Diego |
| *Scarlet Sage (Test 66-6)* | | | | | |
| USS *Herbert J. Thomas* (DD-833) | Destroyer | — | USS *Agerholm* (DD-826) | Destroyer | San Diego, Long Beach |
| *Shady Grove (Test 64-4)* | | | | | |
| USS *Granville S. Hall* (YAG-40) | Auxiliary Ship | Pearl Harbor | USS *Interceptor* (AGR-8) | Auxiliary ship | Bremerton, Washington; Panama Canal Zone; Cuba; Portsmouth, Virginia |
| VMA 214, MAG13 | Attack squadron | — | VMA214, MAG 13 | Attack squadron | — |
| HMM 161, Marine Air Group 13 | Medium helicopter squadron | — | HMM 161, MAG 13 | Medium helicopter squadron | — |
| Light tugs 2080, 2081, 2085, 2086, 2087 | — | — | None selected | — | — |
| *Speckled Start (Test 68-50)* | | | | | |
| USS *Granville S. Hall* (YAG-40) | Auxiliary Ship | Pearl Harbor | USS *Oxford* (ATGR-1) | Auxiliary ship | Philippines, South China Sea |
| Five light tugs (hull numbers not specified) | — | — | None selected | — | — |

NOTE: No personnel were identified for the Flower Drum II test so its units are not represented here.
SOURCE: Adapted from Table 6-2 (IOM, 2007) with additional information from DoD (2015).

## REFERENCES

DoD (Department of Defense). 2015. *Project 112/SHAD fact sheets.* http://www.health.mil/Military-Health-Topics/Health-Readiness/Environmental-Exposures/Project-112-SHAD/Fact-Sheets (accessed October 15, 2015).

IOM (Institute of Medicine). 2007. *Long-term health effects of participation in Project SHAD (Shipboard Hazard and Defense).* Washington, DC: The National Academies Press.

# Appendix F

# Diagnostic Codes Used to Define Health Outcomes

The committee examined the mortality and morbidity experience of Project SHAD (Shipboard Hazard and Defense) veterans and the comparison population using data on cause of death and diagnosis coded in accordance with the *International Classification of Diseases* (ICD). This appendix provides the ICD codes that correspond to the categories of cause of death or diagnosis used in presenting the results of the analyses. Table F-1 presents the codes for the outcome categories for the analyses that tested the committee's literature-based hypotheses regarding exposure to substances used in some SHAD tests. Table F-2 and Table F-3 provide the codes that correspond to the categories used in the exploratory analyses of mortality and morbidity.

**TABLE F-1** International Classification of Disease Codes Used to Define Health Outcomes Examined for Possible Association with Exposure to Specified Substances Used in SHAD Tests

| Exposure and Health Outcome | ICD-9 Codes (2011 version) | ICD-10 Codes (2011 version) |
|---|---|---|
| *Betapropiolactone* | | |
| Cancer (malignant neoplasms), any | 140.x-209.x Malignant neoplasms<br>230.x-234.x Carcinoma in situ<br>V10.xx Personal history of malignant neoplasm | C00-C97 Malignant neoplasms<br>C7A.x Malignant neuroendocrine tumors<br>C7B.x Secondary neuroendocrine tumors<br>D00-D09 In situ neoplasms<br>Z85 Personal history of malignant neoplasm |
| *Coxiella burnetii* | | |
| Endocarditis | 421.x Acute and subacute endocarditis<br>424.9x Endocarditis, valve unspecified<br>424.99 Other endocarditis, valve unspecified | I33 Acute and subacute endocarditis<br>I38 Endocarditis, valve unspecified<br>I39 Endocarditis and heart valve disorders in diseases classified elsewhere |
| Fatigue syndrome | 300.5 Neurasthenia | F48 Other nonpsychotic mental |

| Exposure and Health Outcome | ICD-9 Codes (2011 version) | ICD-10 Codes (2011 version) |
|---|---|---|
| | 780.71 Chronic fatigue syndrome<br>780.79 Other malaise and fatigue | disorders<br>F48.8 Other specified neurotic disorders<br>R53.1 Weakness<br>R53.8 Other malaise and fatigue<br>R53.82 Chronic fatigue, unspecified<br>R53.81 Other malaise<br>R53.83 other fatigue |
| Chronic hepatitis | 571.4x Chronic hepatitis (includes 571.40, 571.41, 571.49)<br>571.42 Autoimmune hepatitis<br>573.3 Hepatitis, unspecified | K73.x Chronic hepatitis, not elsewhere classified<br>K75.4 Autoimmune hepatitis<br>K75.9 Inflammatory liver disease, unspecified (Hepatitis nos) |
| Osteomyelitis | 730.1xx Chronic osteomyelitis<br>730.2xx Unspecified osteomyelitis<br>730.9xx Unspecified infection of bone | M86.6x Other chronic osteomyelitis, unspecified site<br>M86.9 Osteomyelitis, unspecified<br>M86.3x Chronic multifocal osteomyelitis<br>M86.4x Chronic osteomyelitis with draining sinus<br>M86.5x Other chronic hematogenous osteomyelitis<br>M86.8x Other osteomyelitis |
| Vascular infection | 447.6 Arteritis, unspecified | I77.6 Arteritis, unspecified |
| *Escherichia coli* | | |
| Irritable bowel syndrome | 555.x Regional enteritis (Crohn's)<br>556.x Ulcerative enterocolitis<br>558.x Other and unspecified noninfectious gastroenteritis and colitis<br>564.1 Irritable bowel syndrome | K50.x Crohn's disease [regional enteritis]<br>K51.x Ulcerative colitis<br>K52.x Other noninfective gastroenteritis and colitis<br>K58.x Irritable bowel syndrome |
| *Sarin* | | |
| Neurological effects: Central nervous system | 290.xx Dementias<br>323.7x Toxic encephalitis, myelitis, and encephalomyelitis<br>323.8x Other causes of encephalitis, myelitis, and encephalomyelitis<br>327.xx Organic sleep disorders<br>331.xx Other cerebral degenerations (e.g., Alzheimer's disease, frontotemporal dementia, senile degeneration of brain)<br>332.x Parkinson's disease<br>333.0 Other degenerative diseases of | F00.x Dementia in Alzheimer's disease<br>F01.xx Vascular dementia<br>F03.xx Unspecified dementia<br>G92 Toxic encephalopathy<br>G04.8x Other encephalitis, myelitis and encephalomyelitis<br>G47.xx Sleep disorders (organic)<br>G30.x Alzheimer's disease<br>G31.xx Other degenerative diseases of nervous system, not elsewhere classified<br>G20 Parkinson's disease |

| Exposure and Health Outcome | ICD-9 Codes (2011 version) | ICD-10 Codes (2011 version) |
|---|---|---|
| | the basal ganglia<br>333.1 Essential and other specified forms of tremor<br>333.2 Myoclonus<br>333.3 Tics of organic origin<br>333.7 Acquired torsion dystonia<br>333.8 Fragments of torsion dystonia<br>333.9 Other and unspecified extrapyramidal diseases and abnormal movement disorder<br>334.2 Primary cerebellar degeneration<br>334.3 Other cerebellar ataxia<br>334.4 Cerebellar ataxia in diseases classified elsewhere<br>334.8 Other spinocerebellar diseases<br>334.9 Spinocerebellar disease, unspecified<br>335.2x Motor neuron disease (e.g., ALS)<br>336.x Other diseases of spinal cord<br>337.xx Disorders of the autonomic nervous system<br>338.0 Central pain syndrome<br>338.29 Other chronic pain<br>338.4 Chronic pain syndrome<br>339.xx Other Headache Syndromes<br>340 Multiple sclerosis<br>341.xx Other demyelinating diseases of central nervous system<br>342.xx Hemiplegia and hemiparesis<br>344.xx Other paralytic syndromes<br>345.xx Epilepsy and recurrent seizures (excluding 345.6 Infantile spasms)<br>346.xx Migraine<br>347.xx Cataplexy and narcolepsy<br>348.2 Benign intracranial hypertension<br>348.4 Compression of brain<br>348.5 Cerebral edema<br>348.8x Other conditions of brain<br>348.9 Unspecified condition of brain<br>349.2 Disorders of meninges, not elsewhere classified<br>349.8x Other specified disorders of nervous system<br>349.9 Unspecified disorders of nervous system<br>781.xx Symptoms involving nervous | G23.x Other degenerative diseases of basal ganglia<br>G25.0 Essential tremor<br>G25.2 Other specified forms of tremor<br>G25.3 Myoclonus<br>G25.6x Drug induced tics and other tics of organic origin<br>G25.8x Other specified extrapyramidal and movement disorders<br>G25.9 Extrapyramidal and movement disorder, unspecified<br>G24.2x-G24.9x Dystonias<br>G80.3 Athetoid cerebral palsy<br>G11.2 Late-onset cerebellar ataxia<br>G32.81 Cerebellar ataxia in diseases classified elsewhere<br>(Not including hereditary diseases G11.3, G11.8, G11.9)<br>G12.2x Motor Neuron disease<br>G12.8 Other spinal muscular atrophies and related syndromes<br>G12.9 Spinal muscular atrophy, unspecified<br>G95.xx Other diseases of spinal cord<br>G90.xx Disorders of autonomic nervous system<br>G89.0 Central pain syndrome<br>G89.29 Other chronic pain<br>G89.4 Chronic pain syndrome<br>G44.xxx Other headache syndromes<br>G35 Multiple sclerosis<br>G36.x Other acute disseminated demyelination<br>G37.x Other demyelinating diseases of central nervous system<br>G81.xx Hemiplegia<br>G82.xx Paraplegia (paraparesis) and quadriplegia (quadriparesis)<br>G83.xx Other paralytic syndromes<br>G40.xx Epilepsy<br>G43.xxx Migraine<br>G93.2 Benign intracranial hypertension<br>G93.5 Compression of brain<br>G93.6 Cerebral edema<br>G93.8xx Other specified disorders of brain<br>G93.9 Disorder of brain, unspecified<br>G96.1x Disorders of meninges, not |

| Exposure and Health Outcome | ICD-9 Codes (2011 version) | ICD-10 Codes (2011 version) |
|---|---|---|
| | and musculoskeletal systems<br>784.0 Headache<br>780.96 Generalized pain<br>794.0x Nonspecific abnormal results of function study of brain and central nervous system<br>799.5 Signs and symptoms involving cognition | otherwise classified<br>G96.8 Other specified disorders of central nervous system<br>G96.9 Disorder of central nervous system, unspecified<br>G92 Toxic encephalopathy<br>G98.x Other disorders of nervous system not elsewhere classified<br>R25.xxx-R29.xxx Symptoms and signs involving the nervous and musculoskeletal systems<br>R51 Headache<br>R52 Pain, not elsewhere classified<br>R94.0x Abnormal findings of function studies of central nervous system<br>R41.xx Other symptoms and signs involving cognitive functions and awareness<br>R43.x Disturbances of smell and taste |
| Neurological effects: Peripheral nervous system | 350.x Trigeminal nerve disorders<br>351.x Facial nerve disorders<br>352.x Disorders of other cranial nerves<br>353.x Nerve root and plexus disorders<br>354.x Mononeuritis of upper limb and mononeuritis multiplex<br>355.x Mononeuritis of lower limb and unspecified site<br>357.7 Polyneuropathy due to other toxic agents<br>357.9 Unspecified inflammatory and toxic neuropathy<br>358.xx Myoneural disorders<br>359.3 Periodic paralysis<br>359.4 Toxic myopathy<br>359.9 Myopathy, unspecified<br>781.xx Symptoms involving nervous and musculoskeletal systems<br>794.1x Nonspecific abnormal results of function study of peripheral nervous system<br>357.8x Other inflammatory and toxic neuropathy<br>359.5 Myopathy in endocrine diseases classified elsewhere<br>359.6 Symptomatic inflammatory myopathy in diseases classified | G50.x Disorders of trigeminal nerve<br>G51.x Facial nerve disorders<br>G52.x Disorders of other cranial nerves<br>G54.x Nerve root and plexus disorders<br>G55 Nerve root and plexus compressions in diseases classified elsewhere<br>G56.xx Mononeuropathies of upper limb<br>G57.xx Mononeuropathies of lower limb<br>G58.x Other mononeuropathies<br>G62.2 Polyneuropathy due to other toxic agents<br>G61.9 Inflammatory polyneuropathy, unspecified<br>G70.xx Myasthenia gravis and other myoneural disorders<br>G72.3 Periodic paralysis<br>G72.2 Myopathy due to other toxic agents<br>G72.9 Myopathy, unspecified<br>R25.xx-R29.xx Symptoms and signs involving the nervous and musculoskeletal systems<br>R94.1xx Abnormal results of function studies of peripheral nervous system<br>G61.8x Other inflammatory |

| Exposure and Health Outcome | ICD-9 Codes (2011 version) | ICD-10 Codes (2011 version) |
|---|---|---|
| | elsewhere<br>359.7x Inflammatory and immune myopathies, not elsewhere classified | polyneuropathies<br>G62.8 Other specified polyneuropathies<br>G72.4x Inflammatory myopathy, not elsewhere classified<br>G64 Other disorders of peripheral nervous system |
| Neurological effects: Hearing loss | 389.xx Hearing loss<br>385.0x Tympanosclerosis<br>385.1x Adhesive middle ear disease<br>385.2x Other acquired abnormality of ear ossicles<br>387.x Otosclerosis<br>388.xx Other disorders of ear | H90.xx Conductive and sensorineural hearing loss<br>H91.xx Other hearing loss<br>H74.0x Tympanosclerosis<br>H74.1x Adhesive middle ear disease<br>H74.3x Other acquired abnormalities of ear ossicles<br>H80.xx Otosclerosis<br>H93.xxx-H94.xxx Other disorders of ear |
| Psychological symptoms | 293.xx Transient mental disorders due to conditions classified elsewhere<br>294.xx Persistent mental disorders due to conditions classified elsewhere<br>295.xx Schizophrenic disorders<br>296.xx Episodic mood disorders<br>297.x Delusional disorders<br>298.x Other nonorganic psychoses<br>300.xx Anxiety, dissociative and somatoform disorders<br>301.xx Personality disorders<br>303.xx Alcohol dependence syndrome<br>304.xx Drug dependence<br>305.xx Nondependent abuse of drugs<br>306.xx Physiological malfunction arising from mental factors<br>307.xx Special symptoms or syndromes not elsewhere classified (e.g., sleep, eating, tics)<br>309.xx Adjustment reaction<br>311 Depressive disorder, not elsewhere classified<br>312.xx Disturbance of conduct not elsewhere classified<br>316 Psychic factors associated with diseases classified elsewhere<br>797 Senility without mention of psychosis<br>799.2x Nervousness<br>799.3 Debility, unspecified<br>799.5 Signs and symptoms involving | F02.8 Dementia in other specified diseases classified elsewhere<br>F03 Unspecified dementia<br>F04 Organic amnesic syndrome, not induced by alcohol and other psychoactive substances<br>F05 Delirium not induced by alcohol and other psychoactive substances<br>F06 Other mental disorders due to brain damage and dysfunction and to physical disease<br>F07 Personality and behavioral disorders due to brain disease, damage, and dysfunction<br>F09 Unspecified organic or symptomatic mental disorder<br>F10-F19 Mental and behavioral disorders due to psychoactive substance use<br>F20-F29 Schizophrenia, schizotypal and delusional disorders<br>F30-39 Mood [affective] disorders<br>F40-48 Neurotic, stress-related and somatoform disorders<br>F50-59 Behavioral syndromes associated with physiological disturbances and physical factors<br>F60 Specific personality disorders<br>F61 Mixed and other personality disorders<br>R54 Senility (without mention of |

| Exposure and Health Outcome | ICD-9 Codes (2011 version) | ICD-10 Codes (2011 version) |
|---|---|---|
| | cognition<br>308.x Acute reaction to stress | psychosis)<br>R45.0 Nervousness<br>R53 Malaise and fatigue<br>R41 Other symptoms and signs involving cognitive functions and awareness |
| *Staphylococcal enterotoxin type B* | | |
| Asthma | 493 Asthma (includes 493.x, 493.xx) | J45.xx Asthma |
| Graves' disease | 242.xx Thyrotoxicosis with or without goiter | E05.xx Thyrotoxicosis (includes Graves' disease) |
| Multiple sclerosis | 340 Multiple sclerosis | G35 Multiple sclerosis |
| Rheumatoid arthritis: Broad definition | 714.0 Rheumatoid arthritis<br>714.1 Felty's syndrome<br>714.2 Other rheumatoid arthritis with visceral or systemic involvement<br>715.xx Osteoarthrosis and allied disorders<br>720.0 Ankylosing spondylitis<br>721.x Spondylosis | M05.xxx Rheumatoid arthritis with rheumatoid factor<br>M06.xx Other rheumatoid arthritis<br>M15.xxx Polyosteoarthritis<br>M16.xxx Osteoarthritis of hip<br>M17.xxx Osteoarthritis of knee<br>M18.xxx Osteoarthritis of first carpometacarpal joint<br>M19.xxx Other and unspecified osteoarthritis<br>M45.xxx Ankylosing spondylitis<br>M47.xxx Spondylosis<br>M48.xxx Other spondylopathies |
| Rheumatoid arthritis: Narrow definition | 714.0 Rheumatoid arthritis<br>714.1 Felty's syndrome<br>714.2 Other rheumatoid arthritis with visceral or systemic involvement<br>720.0 Ankylosing spondylitis | M05.xxx Rheumatoid arthritis with rheumatoid factor<br>M06.xxx Other rheumatoid arthritis<br>M45.xxx Ankylosing spondylitis |
| *Zinc cadmium sulfide* | | |
| Lung cancer | 162.2, 162.3, 162.4, 162.5, 162.8, 162.9 Malignant neoplasm of bronchus or lung (excluding 162.0 Malignant neoplasm of trachea)<br>231.2 Carcinoma in situ of respiratory system<br>V10.11 personal history of malignant neoplasm of bronchus or lung | C34.xx Malignant neoplasm of bronchus and lung<br>D02.20 Carcinoma in situ of bronchus and lung<br>Z85.11x Personal history of malignant neoplasm of trachea, bronchus and lung |
| Chronic kidney disease: Broad definition | 403.xx (includes stages I-IV)<br>404.xx Hypertensive heart and chronic kidney disease, stage V or ESRD | I12 xx (includes I12.9 stage I-IV)<br>I13xx Hypertensive heart and chronic kidney disease or end stage renal |

| Exposure and Health Outcome | ICD-9 Codes (2011 version) | ICD-10 Codes (2011 version) |
|---|---|---|
| | 440.1 Atherosclerosis of renal artery<br>442.1 Aneurysm of renal artery<br>572.4 Hepatorenal syndrome<br>580.xx Acute glomerulonephritis<br>581.xx Nephrotic syndrome<br>582.xx Chronic glomerulonephritis<br>583.xx Nephritis and nephropathy not specified as acute or chronic<br>584.x Acute kidney failure)<br>585.x Chronic kidney disease<br>586 Renal failure, unspecified<br>587 Renal sclerosis, unspecified<br>588.xx Disorders resulting from impaired renal function<br>591 Hydronephrosis<br>794.4 Nonspecific abnormal results of kidney function study<br>249.4x Secondary diabetes mellitus with renal manifestations<br>250.4x Diabetes with renal manifestations<br>271.4 Renal glycosuria<br>274.10 Gout nephropathy<br>283.11 Hemolytic uremic syndrome<br>589.x Small kidney of unknown origin | disease (includes stage I-IV and V)<br>I70.1 Atherosclerosis of renal artery<br>I72.2 Aneurysm of renal artery<br>K76.7 Hepatorenal syndrome<br>N00-N06, N08 Glomerular diseases (excluding N07 hereditary nephropathy, nos)<br>N17 Acute renal failure<br>N18 Chronic kidney disease<br>N19 Unspecified kidney failure<br>N26 Unspecified contracted kidney<br>N25 Disorders resulting from impaired renal tubular function<br>N13.1, 13.2, 13.3 Hydronephrosis<br>R94.4 Abnormal results of kidney function studies<br>E08.22, E09.22, E10.22, E11.22<br>E13.22 diabetic chronic kidney disease<br>M10.3x Gout due to renal impairment, unspecified site<br>D59.3 Hemolytic-uremic syndrome<br>N27 Small kidney of unknown cause |
| Chronic kidney disease: Narrow definition | 440.1 Atherosclerosis of renal artery<br>581.xx Nephrotic syndrome<br>582.xx Chronic glomerulonephritis<br>583.xx Nephritis and nephropathy not specified as acute or chronic<br>585.x Chronic kidney disease<br>586 Renal failure, unspecified<br>587 Renal sclerosis, unspecified<br>588.xx Disorders resulting from impaired renal function<br>794.4 Nonspecific abnormal results of kidney function study<br>580.xx Acute glomerulonephritis<br>584.x Acute kidney failure<br>589.x Small kidney of unknown origin | I70.1 Atherosclerosis of renal artery<br>N04 Nephrotic syndrome<br>N03 Chronic nephritic syndrome<br>N05 Unspecified nephritic syndrome<br>N18 Chronic kidney disease<br>N19 Unspecified kidney failure<br>N26 Unspecified contracted kidney<br>N25 Disorders resulting from impaired renal tubular function<br>R94.4 Abnormal results of kidney function studies<br>N00 Acute nephritic syndrome<br>N17 Acute Renal failure<br>N27 Small kidney of unknown cause |

NOTE: An x in a code indicates that all versions of the code category preceding the x are included. For example, a code shown as 123.x indicates that the category includes instances of outcomes coded as 123.0, 123.1, . . ., or 123.9. An xx entry indicates a two-digit range of codes (e.g., 123.00, 123.01, etc.).

**TABLE F-2** Broad Categories of Underlying Cause of Death and the Corresponding Codes from the *International Classification of Diseases*

| Cause of Death | ICD-9 (2011 ICD-9 CM) | ICD-10 Codes |
|---|---|---|
| Cancer (malignant neoplasms), any | 140-209, V10 | C00-C97, Z85 |
| Cardiovascular disease [Circulatory disease] | 390-459 | I00-I99 |
| *Ischemic heart disease* | *410-414* | *I20-I25* |
| *Other heart disease* | *390-409, 415-459* | *I00-I19, I26-I99* |
| Respiratory disease | 460-519 | J00-J99 |
| Endocrine and metabolic diseases | 240-279 | E00-E90 |
| Infectious diseases | 001-139 | A00-B99 |
| Injury/external causes | 800-959, E codes 800-999 | S00-T98, V01-X84 |
| Neurocognitive problems | 290-319, 320-327 | F00-F99, G00-G09 |

**TABLE F-3** Broad Categories of Diagnoses Received from Inpatient or Outpatient Medical Care and the Corresponding Codes from the *International Classification of Diseases*, Ninth Revision

| Diagnostic Categories | ICD-9 (2011 ICD-9 CM) |
|---|---|
| Infectious diseases | 001-139 |
| Cancer (neoplasms, including malignant, benign, in situ) | 140-209, 210-229, 230-234, 235-238, 239-239, V10.xx |
| Endocrine and metabolic diseases | 240-279 |
| Diseases of the blood and blood-forming organs | 280-289 |
| Mental disorders | 290-319 |
| Nervous system and sense organs | 320-389 |
| Circulatory disease | 390-459 |
| *Ischemic heart disease* | *410-414* |
| *Other heart disease* | *390-409, 415-459* |
| Respiratory disease | 460-519 |
| Digestive disease | 520-579 |
| Genitourinary disease | 580-629 |
| Skin disease | 680-709 |
| Musculoskeletal disease | 710-739 |
| Symptoms, signs and abnormal clinical and laboratory findings, not elsewhere classified | 780-799 |
| Injury | 800-959, E codes 800-999 |
| Neurocognitive problems | 290-319, 320-327 |

NOTES: Claims criteria: At least 1 inpatient, or 2 HOP or Carrier claims with diagnosis codes during the 1-year period; codes have to be on 2 different days. HHA = home health agency; HOP = hospital outpatient.